Drug-Free Arthritis

To order additional copies, please contact us at:
Charo Publishing
85 Bronson Avenue, Suite 504
Ottawa, ON, Canada K1R 6G7
613-237-3580
www.CharlesSeems.com

CHARLES SEEMS

DRUG-FREE ARTHRITIS
Secrets to Successful Living

2006

Drug-Free Arthritis

TABLE OF CONTENTS

To My Late Mother Who Taught Me By Word And By Example That Hard Work, Passion And Being True To Me Would Lead To A Life Of Health And Success.

To The Late Wally Coulombe, My Mentor In Youth, Who Took The Time To Share His Wisdom And To Care For Me In Ways Only A True Friend Can.

To Robert Labine Jr., My Spouse, Who Has Been My Steadfast Support And Greatest Fan.

To Marie Lapointe And Cyanna Mitchell, Whose Constant Love And Friendship Over The Years Have Given Me Courage To Face My Greatest Fears.

To Françoise Plourde And Brian Tardiff For Being There In My Time Of Need.

To Louise Davignon For Believing In Me And The Value Of This Book.

To My Cousin Lise (Aubé) Mackenzie, Whose Care And Compassion For The Sick And Elderly Are What Makes Her Such A Special Person.

And Finally, To My Dear Friends Jim Taylor And Brian Kuerze Of Wallingford, Connecticut, Whose Personal Challenges And Successes Have Inspired Me Beyond Belief.

PREAMBLE

D o the thing you fear and the death of fear is certain."[1] This book is about dealing with chronic pain. This book is also about success. It is not meant to replace the sound advice given by medical professionals. Rather, it is a compendium of thoughts, ideas, anecdotes, outlooks, quotes, recommendations, and even some recipes to help you build a better pain management strategy. Although geared toward arthritis sufferers, the common sense approach to healthy living that emerges from the following pages is sure to benefit anyone who is concerned about living better and more successfully.

Who knows how long it will be before a cure for arthritis is found? In the interim, we are inundated with new drugs coming on the market at an unprecedented pace. Although these may offer some temporary relief, there is little research on the prolonged use of drugs and its impact on the human body. A growing number of people are turning to alternative therapies that provide relief from pain without any side effects. Alternative therapies include acupuncture, acupressure, yoga, plants, and herbs. As stated so simply by Dr. D.C. Jarvis in his 1958 book *Folk Medicine: A New England almanac of natural health care from a noted Vermont country doctor*, "Nature opened the first drug store. Primitive man and the animals use its stock of plants and herbs to avoid disease and to remain health and vigorous."

The notion that I could rid myself of arthritic pain and stay away from drugs altogether came from a story I found in the above noted book. "One day a farmer dropped in at the office to report on his arthritis. He said that before taking ten teaspoonfuls of apple cider vinegar to a glass of water with each meal he had lameness in all the joints of his body. The first day after he began taking the mixture, his lameness was 20 per cent better and there was still more improvement on the second day. By the fourth he estimated a 50 per cent improvement, and at the end of a month a 75 per cent improvement. In addition to the lameness he had had pain in the joints, but that cleared up as the lameness lessened. Finally the pain cleared up altogether, including pain in the back of the head and neck."

Drug companies are not interested in curing people. These companies exist for the purpose of making money. The more pills we buy, the more money they make. New product advertisements usually contain a list of side effects that one might expect. However, there is no easy way to find out how the compounding of medication—taking several drugs at the same time—will impact one's body. Whether using one or more drugs, the full and long term effects of drug use are seldom, if ever, known at the outset.

Increasingly, people are finding solutions to their medical problems without resorting to drugs. This is not to say that drugs don't have a place in a person's medical treatment. For a person whose condition is out of control or very severe, drugs may be the best or only way to fight against a disease. Delaying the use of drugs, where possible, is what I advocated in this book.

Responding to what ails us, we naturally turn to topical solutions that address our physical needs. That is why taking medication which offers a quick remedy or masks symptoms is a preferred option. Yet there are many other options available to us. For centuries, aboriginal and oriental societies have relied on other forms of medication. In recent decades, we have borrowed from Eastern medicine to supplement our pain management options. Natural healing based on the wise and informed use of ingredients found in various natural habitats has provided alternatives worth investigating.

Over the years, I have come to the conclusion that pain management and prevention goes way beyond finding solutions to immediate concerns. It has become increasingly clear to me that lifestyle choices directly impact our physical condition. In addition to the physical aspects of life, I have found that the intellectual, emotional, and spiritual dimensions have an important part to play in well-being. If managed properly, a balanced lifestyle can lead to a healthy and positive outcome. It can offer new hope as preventive actions will certainly minimize degenerative illnesses such as arthritis. In my opinion, this balanced lifestyle should take the form a 'holistic' approach to living.

How you think affects how you feel. When stressed or depressed, your body takes a beating. If you do not manage your stress or get help for your depression, you will soon begin to feel ill, which in turn will affect your morale. It's a vicious cycle that is hard to break. A holistic approach to life provides you with a better chance of maintaining a drug-free existence for as long as possible.

Since one's physical health is largely dependant on mental health, I looked for models to emulate. First I noticed that some people are the picture of physical health but lack the knowledge or skills to ensure a good life. Then I observed those whose mental agility is awesome despite obvious physical problems or ailments. Later I found a small number of people who, it seemed, had struck just the right balance of brawn and brain development. To my amazement, these well-adjusted individuals allowed for a compartmentalization of their lives and took time to nurture each of the elements of a holistic life. Their approach is based on paying attention to all facets of living, which include proper eating, sufficient rest, regular physical activity, avoidance of irritants (foods or otherwise), solid values, commitment, and realistic life perspectives.

In all cases, I found these individuals to be quite successful. I concluded that there is a link between well-being and success. I will use the term 'success' to define those individuals who have achieved a measure of balance in what they do. Finding one's reason or passion in life is key to achieving this balance, but more on this topic later.

In reading this book, you will wonder if in fact it deals more with success than arthritis. To a large extent, that is true. Living a 'drug-free arthritis' lifestyle is a first step towards success and this book will reveal many other secrets that will enhance your well-being to a point where your arthritis may be reduced to infrequent annoying stiffness, which you can easily manage.

Few people would ever know that I have arthritis since I have no highly-visible symptoms. The one exception, if you looked closely, is that my head has a reduced range. When turning my head to the left, I can only go about 40 degrees. The vast majority of people are shocked when they find out that I've had arthritis for more than thirty-five years. What I don't tell them is what I do to remain healthy. This is the purpose of this book. As I have been both lucky and successful, people I meet are curious to know what I have done and what I do now to maintain such a level of health and success. I've attempted to enlighten a few close friends but have found it very tedious to explain as my approaches are intertwined. It's like a giant puzzle with many pieces. Once all the pieces are together, then you see the whole picture.

I will first start by describing what the whole picture, or puzzle, looks like and then I'll discuss each piece separately. The picture is 'success'. My definition of success is based on realistic life expectations and perspectives.

Ever wondered how successful people reach success? Success is both doing and being. It's as much taking appropriate steps to succeed as it is adopting an attitude of 'I must, I can, I will'. The key to success is self-determination. People who really want to succeed and are ready to work towards it have a much greater chance of getting there than those who simply wish it. "To them, it doesn't matter how hard you try or how talented you are, being successful is like winning the lottery; it's all a matter of luck. With this attitude, it hardly makes sense to work hard or be dedicated to a dream or goal."[2] My goal is to live drug-free for as long as I can. The more I work at it, the better the chance I will have at success.

There are no accidents in life; things happen for a reason. When things don't go the way you had planned them, the reasons may not be immediately clear. It may take weeks or months, and in some cases years, before you fully understand why certain events have taken place. Looking back and analyzing the circumstances surrounding a particular event can help you understand the lesson you needed to learn.

In the movie 'The Sound of Music', Sister Maria is bound and determined to become a nun. Yet her life takes an unexpected turn after she becomes the governess to Captain von Trapp's children. Although unplanned events in your life may not be as dramatic as was the case with Sister Maria, they happen for a reason. Do you bother to look back and try to find the lessons to be learned?

When something unplanned or unexpected occurs, it may send you in a different direction than the road you had anticipated taking. Even the best-laid plans can be dismissed as you are challenged in other directions. In trying to reassure Sister Maria, Mother Superior responded with all the maternal instinct she could muster: "My child, when the Lord closes a door, somewhere he opens a window." Mother Superior was convinced that the road to success can take many turns. Some of these will undoubtedly leave you wondering if your goals are being compromised. You simply have to believe that what is happening to you is in your best interest.

Driving back from the cottage, there are times when I get annoyed as the traffic comes to a halt. I think to myself: "what a waste of time" or "I'm going to be late". The last time the traffic was slow, I arrived on the scene of a major accident, just minutes after the crash. I couldn't help but wonder what would have happened had the traffic been going its normal speed. Would I have been involved in that accident? "There but for the grace of God go I," I think to myself and resolve to accept what I can't change.

Other times when I am delayed for whatever reason, I'm surprised that my lateness is rewarded by a chance meeting with someone who I wanted to see or who wanted to see me. These opportunities are not to be missed. Whether or not you believe in fate is a matter of personal choice. I would rather believe that I have some control over my destiny but not all the time.

Having said this, I firmly believe that there are no errors or mistakes in life but rather difficulties, setbacks, and challenges. One may argue that this is simply a question of semantics, and I agree in part. However, I would rather see the glass as half full as opposed to half empty. Successful people shy away from negative things, people and events. When confronted by a difficulty or setback, they ask themselves these questions: "What did I do right?" and "What could have I done differently?"

For people living with arthritis, leading a successful life requires a greater degree a determination than is otherwise required. Having made a choice of drug-free living, arthritis sufferers need to find ways and means to reduce or eliminate pain through appropriate activities and approaches. It is these activities and approaches, if properly followed, that will sustain a drug-free effort over time. In this book, I will discuss, at great length, a whole gamut of personal and not-so-personal secrets to success and pain free living.

The more successes I have, the easier it is to remain drug-free. The happier I am, the more endorphins are produced by my body and consequently the less likely I will experience pain.

Warning: If you are dependant on drugs, before acting on any of the suggestions contained herein, you should consult your doctor or a rheumatologist familiar with your case. Weaning oneself off of drugs, particularly when a specific combination of drug therapies provides much needed relief, can be a long process and should be done only under the guidance of a medical authority.

"If a man advances confidently in the direction of his dreams, he will experience a success unknown in common times."[3]

INTRODUCTION

To understand the degree of success I have had, you need to know a bit about myself and my trials and tribulations thus far. I am well aware that many have suffered much more than I. While it is difficult to compare one person to another when it comes to diseases, I can honestly say that the secrets I share with you in this book have helped me immensely. Had it not been for solutions found by design or sheer luck, I would not likely have written this book since I would most certainly be focusing on my illness.

I was only eighteen when the dreaded diagnosis of Ankylosing Spondylitis was confirmed by my family doctor. Ankylosing Spondylitis—or 'AS', as it is known in the medical community—was once considered a rare, predominantly male disease that progresses relentlessly to spinal fusion. AS belongs to the arthritis family and may spread to other parts of the body. Arthritis is a family of diseases including osteo—and rheumatoid arthritis, multiple sclerosis, lupus, juvenile arthritis, and scleroderma. Genetic predispositions, viruses, lifestyle, and injury all play a role in joint inflammation. Whatever the cause, one in six North Americans have arthritis of some type.

Although discovering arthritis should not have come as a big surprise to me, I was nonetheless annoyed at having to accept that my life would be permanently affected by chronic pain and stiffness.

While growing up, I had witnessed the ravages of AS

on my mother and a few of her brothers. It wasn't difficult to see that, at times, on some days, she was going through excruciating pain. She did take a number of pills for her arthritis but it was hard to tell whether any of them had an effect. Mother claimed that regular rest, exercise, and yoga made her feel better. Through her bouts of pain, I felt helpless despite all I could do to ease her workload. In many ways, it was her strength to carry on despite this burden that made me realize that one could overcome such adversity. I guess, in my mind, my mother was a success.

In the early fall of 1970, I knew that success for me would require that I commit myself to a life of medical uncertainty coupled with a fear of growing old and worn out 'before my time'. "Time is of the essence", I repeated to remind myself that if I was going to achieve success, I didn't have a minute to lose. Where does one begin?

For the following few years, I busied myself with post-secondary education. After many trials and tribulations, I finally obtained a university degree, a recognition that was, at the time, most important to me. I needed to know that despite the years of pain and limping to get to classes, I could achieve goals just like anybody else. With my credentials in hand, I was now ready to move on with my life in pursuit of my dreams. The lure of the big city was too much to resist, so I packed my meager belongings and went west.

Few people in their early twenties have reason to worry about pain and discomfort. Not so for me. At that point in my life, I had grown accustomed to the fact that my body was not able to withstand the types of blows one gets from sports such as downhill skiing or soccer. Not that I was sports-minded but I felt deprived from being able to participate. I preferred not taking any chances that would or could worsen my condition. I was doing relatively well and could manage the AS.

However, in times of stress, I could not keep the AS under control. Life in the fast lane in the metropolis was taking its toll. My family doctor suggested that I meet with a rheumatologist to reconfirm the AS and to see what medical advances might benefit me. After a thorough analysis, the rheumatologist turned to me and with a sad face announced that, in her opinion, I would be in a wheelchair by the time I reached forty.

What about this successful life I had planned on? Would I be able to make my mark on the world or would I be sentenced to a life of misery? "Oh, we have wonderful drugs that can help you," she replied as she noticed my eyes tear up. I took the prescription and walked out of her office vowing that I would never return to see her and that I would not be in a wheelchair at forty, damn it!

From that day on, my journey to success took on a whole new meaning. It is in times of deep hurt or major setback that one is able to face the music in a way that may not otherwise be possible. I was determined that AS would not get the better of me although I knew then, as I do now, that by living a balanced life, I could be successful to the degree I wanted.

As the disease progressed, so did the pain and stiffness. I limped, I cried, I took pain killers and anti-inflammation drugs. As a degenerative disease, AS hits harder as the years go by. Work was stressful. Relationships were made difficult. I came close to ending it all one winter evening as I sat in the bath tub with scalding water up to my neck. I simply couldn't sleep because of the pain and the most comfortable place for me was in very warm water. I certainly didn't want to sleep in the tub and I was tired and exhausted having spent countless nights trying to get some relief. Should I end my life, my misery? Could there possibly be other ways of reducing the pain? I answered 'no' to the first question and 'yes' to the second question without giving it much thought. I went back to bed and cried myself to sleep. The answers would come, I thought. I just needed to believe in fate.

Thirty-two years after the first AS diagnosis and ten years after the dreaded forty-year marker, I am as healthy as can be expected. The closest I got to being confined to a wheelchair was the day I left the hospital following cataract surgery. Over the years, the AS had spread to my eyes. My right eye suffered a series of uveitis attacks and a cataract had developed. I was fortunate in that I lived close to the Ottawa Eye Institute, where Dr. William Hodge attends to patients from far and wide.

Uveitis can be described as inflammation of the uvea. My first attack of uveitis was misdiagnosed as pinkeye. By the time I came to the attention of highly specialized ophthalmologists who immediately recognized the condition, the flare-up had reached a 3.5 out of a four rating. With appropriate medication, we were able to get the situation under control. Many other bouts of uveitis followed and during one of the most severe episodes, when immediate medication was critical in order to avoid future eyesight damage, I was injected with steroids. It sounds worse than it actually was. It is when the freezing starts to fade away that the discomfort takes hold of you. Thankfully, uveitis attacks start to diminish greatly in intensity and frequency by the age of fifty.

AS may not be as life-altering as cancer; however, in my case, it was the catalyst that led me to look at life in a different way than most. What many people take for granted, I took seriously as I sensed that if I could manage this disease, perhaps my purpose on earth would be revealed.

On the day I turned fifty, I attended a meeting of professional speakers in Ottawa, Ontario, Canada. That two-and-a-half-hour meeting brought much perspective to my life and helped me to further refine my purpose. It was on the beautiful Saturday morning of September 14, 2002, that I understood the need to share my story using my God-given talents of writing and speaking. I have long advocated that we all have choices in life. Doing nothing is an option. But in my case, my choices and options were before me and I needed to get moving.

A year later at a Canadian Association of Professional Speakers (CAPS) meeting, in September 2003, ironically again on a beautiful Saturday morning, I listened to a keynote address by Mark Leblanc, an internationally-acclaimed speaker, who talked about *small business success*. Mark had many wonderful messages, but one in particular hit home. It was targeted to the perfectionists in the audience. He used the expression 'better done that perfect'. Those four words, as simple as they are, were enough to move me to continue work on this book. After all, how could I write about success if I did not have the nerve to get down to the task and do it? Success doesn't come on a silver platter. Hors d'oeuvres maybe!

Christopher Morley[4] was on the right track when he wrote, "There is only one success—to be able to spend your life in your own way." I have finally found the way I want to live my life. And if in reading the following chapters, you are inspired by just one tiny idea or thought, then all the hours and sweat expended writing this book will have been worth it. If the contents of this book inspire you to take action and improve your health, I will have reached a personal goal.

I have deliberately kept this book short so that it may be read quickly and so that no time is lost in starting to apply the secrets contained herein.

Before you start, consider the following facts from the Arthritis Foundation:

The perceptions about arthritis vary, but the numbers don't lie:

- Arthritis is America's number one cause of disability
- 66 million Americans have arthritis and chronic joint symptoms
- 300,000 people with arthritis are children
- Arthritis costs the US economy nearly $86.2 billion annually in lost wages
- There are more than 100 forms of arthritis

"All you need in this life is ignorance and confidence, and then success is sure."[5]

WHAT IS SUCCESS?

Anyone who deals with chronic pain will tell you that overcoming the challenges associated with constant discomfort and pain wears you down and makes for difficult living. It is hard to focus on achievements when you are concerned about getting through the day. However, the link between pain and success may be closer than you think. Focusing on small successes each day will eventually make an impact. In a holistic approach to life, a person needs to start small and build as time goes on. Each small successful step encourages you to take further action on a physical or emotional level. The more you succeed, the less impact pain will have on your life. The stronghold pain has had on your life can and will be diminished to the extent that you focus on getting your life in order and on being successful.

Nothing succeeds like success. But what is success? Success means different things to different people. Webster's Dictionary defines success as "the accomplishment of what is desired or aimed at; attainment of wealth, fame, prosperity, etc." The majority of us focus is on the second part of the definition. For many, wealth, if not fame, is the cornerstone of success.

The outcome of success is twofold: tangible results and intangible results. Obviously, the tangible results are what most people point to when referring to a successful person. Having an above average amount of wealth (money, stocks, bonds, etc.), or possessions (cars, boats, residences, etc.) makes a person stand out from the crowd. On the other hand, intangible results draw less attention. These include recognition, education, happiness, and so forth.

In today's world, success is most often measured by the degree of a person's wealth or fame. There are numerous examples of people who have neither wealth nor fame but who are extremely successful. At the other end of the spectrum are those who have wealth and fame but are still not happy with their lives.

Before attempting to further define what success is, it would be helpful to look at what it is not. Although the dictionary gives us a sense of what success is commonly held to mean, you can still succeed without having accumulated large sums of money and fame. In fact, much can be said about the negative side of wealth and fame. That is not to say that having money or fame is detrimental to your well-being. Most everyone would agree that having an adequate supply of money makes life easier. Money is certainly a commodity which we all need. How much of it you need will depend on your desire and aspirations.

But wealth is not just about money. You can be wealthy in many other ways. Having what you need or desire is all the wealth needed. The decision is yours to make. Throughout my travels, I have always been struck by the degree of happiness I have witnessed in some of the poorest corners of the world. What have they learned that we have overlooked or neglected? Is their happiness a sign of success?

Achieving success corresponds to the highest level of needs as described in Clayton Alderfer's ERG theory. Taking Maslow's hierarchy of needs one step further, Alderfer maps outs three levels of need:

—Existence: Physiological and safety needs
—Relatedness: Social and external esteem needs
—Growth: Self-actualization and internal esteem needs

Unlike Maslow's model, the ERG theory is hierarchical. Existence needs prevail over relatedness, which has priority over growth.

Happiness can occur at all three levels. The higher one wants to move up, the more difficult the challenges will be and happiness may be affected. To forsake happiness for success at all costs may seem hardly worth the trouble. At the growth level, a person is looking to achieve self-actualization. Self-actualization is the quest for one's full potential as a person. This need is never fully satisfied; as one grows psychologically there are always new opportunities to continue to grow. Self-actualized people tend to have needs such as truth, justice, wisdom, and meaning. Giving meaning to your life through enjoyable work experiences that make a positive difference in the lives of others is self-actualization. In doing so, presumably, you would be happy, successful, and living the life that you were meant to live.

How *you* define success is all that is important. All too often, people define success based on values that are not necessarily theirs. In the western world, we are constantly fed a diet of rags to riches stories through various sources such as the film industry, television, sports and the Internet. What you see and what you are told about stars and celebrities is usually focused on glamour.

People are overly-concerned and some even consumed by what their neighbors might say or think. You really can't worry about what others think or you'll never do anything original and never be authentic. Worrying about what others think can get in the way of a person's ability to clearly define for themselves how high the success bar is placed. Do you need the latest toys to be happy? Can you make do with less? Can you live with 'less than perfect', 'less than brand new'? The answer is definitely yes. However, would you? Why not? Societal values are changing. Perhaps the pendulum has swung as far as it could go. It is time to come back to a saner way of life.

Success in my opinion is a state of being—a journey—and not an accumulation of possessions which will need to be disposed of at the end of your life. Success is all about being comfortable with yourself and the activities that make up your daily life. Success is also having the degree of health you need to do the things you want. Finally, success also means having the resources—the money—to meet your basic needs as well as your desires.

Does age have anything to do with success? Maybe! What is important is that one can be successful at any age. It's simply a matter of desire. Having traveled to many parts of the world, I have concluded that it is human nature to want to be successful. I have seen highly successful people in the dark corners of Asia, in the cold regions of Scandinavia, in the peasant towns of South America, and in the hot cities of Egypt. Everywhere I've traveled, what has impressed me most is people's ability to succeed even in conditions that we, in North America, would find deplorable.

I've also learned that successful people make it happen. As I have learned more on the topic of success, I have been drawn to different types of people expressing or living their successes in very different ways. What I have come away with is that everyone can succeed given the right tools, the right directions, the right attitudes, and a desire to do so.

Success depends on your determination, your motivation, your will power and persistence. To reach success and gain the habits you want to have, to acquire the skills you desire, you absolutely must change the way you think. To create success that feels as normal as it does for the people you've been in awe of your whole life, you must be ready to commit to refocusing toward positive thinking and doing. This means acquiring the skills to turn negative thoughts and images into self-empowering energies.

Paradoxically, the single most important element of success is giving. Giving is both sharing and receiving. When you give of yourself, be it time, advice, money, or ideas, it all comes back to you in spades. You may have heard the expression that 'what goes around comes around'. It is often used to warn people that by doing harm to others harm will come to them. On the positive side, by helping others, the favor will be returned by the least likely of all. For many people, the concept of giving is only acceptable if the person you gave to will be the one who comes to your rescue in your time of need. However, that person may not have what you require when you require it. Don't be too surprised when the help comes from an unexpected party.

Part of being successful is being true to yourself. Regardless of your beliefs, religious or otherwise, being real should dominate your list of goals. We live in a world of make-believe where blemishes are unwanted and any form of fakery is acceptable. We airbrush out of lives those parts that we would prefer others not to see. We spend so much time worrying about what others might see or think that we forget about being ourselves. Being true to yourself means accepting yourself as you are and working to improve those areas that you wish to change. If you want to be successful, you need to start at the very core of your being. Have you ever noticed how truly successful people radiate? Ever wonder why? The answer is simple. They have understood that to be successful you have to be yourself.

While I was growing up, my mother tried to pass that message on to me. The way she did it made a profound impact on me. When the song "I've got to be me" played on the radio, she made a point of singing along and looking at me straight in the eyes. It was as if she knew that part of my challenges in life would be just that: accepting myself the way I am. I was perhaps too inexperienced to see that it also meant living with arthritis. Later on, that same message was brought back to me with another song entitled "I am what I am." Without going into the lyrics of these songs, the mere titles should be food for thought.

Success...

"To laugh often and love much;

to win the respect of intelligent persons and the affection of children;

to earn the approbation of honest citizens and endure the betrayal of false friends;

to appreciate beauty;

to find the best in others;

to give of one's self;

to leave the world a bit better,

whether by a healthy child,

a garden patch or a redeemed social condition;

to have played and laughed with enthusiasm and sung with exultation;

to know that even one life has breathed easier because you have lived—

this is to have succeeded."

Ralph Waldo Emerson

GETTING STARTED

Taking concrete action to improve your situation will help you move away from a life of arthritic pain and discomfort. Each and every step is important in turning your life around. Unless you are committed to action on a daily basis, any progress you make will be lost in a matter of days. If success is your goal, then you should be prepared to face the daily challenges required to reduce or eliminate pain while you take concrete action to set objectives and make plans for getting what you want out of life. Success and healthy living depend on you. Some successes will be easy while other will test your limits.

Success starts on the first day of your life. The moment you step outside your Mother's placenta, you begin a long journey fraught with challenges the first of which you have already overcome. You are alive and well and should no further complications occur, you complete a full day of living. That is a significant step. People take these accomplishments with a grain of salt as medical advances have almost erased the possibility of things going wrong within the first twenty-four hours of our lives. How lucky we are!

Your journey through life is a succession of challenges, some of which you will be able to overcome on the first try while others will require more time and patience. The child who starts to crawl will eventually be able to stand and walk a short distance. As soon as this challenge is in the past, the child will move forward to bigger and greater feats. At that young age, there is so much to learn, so much to conquer that success is possible on a daily basis. By the time a newborn celebrates a second birthday, the challenges become a bit more difficult. Seeing another child attempt and succeed walking up a set of stairs, for example, is enough to challenge a child to do likewise and try to succeed on the first attempt. Rarely is this possible as it requires a degree of balance and confidence that comes with time. Frustration sets in followed by crying spells and more attempts till one day, success comes. Now that the toddler has made it up the stairs, coming back down presents a whole new set of challenges and risks. The process of trial and error is used and eventually the toddler is able to begin the practice needed to meet this newest test of strength and personality.

The process of learning that occurs through multiple attempts at reaching a goal is repeated throughout life. Very few could declare that they were successful on a first attempt to meet a specific goal. You observe, you read, you study, and then perhaps you feel ready to give something a try. Driving a car, for example, although not a very difficult challenge, requires you to examine how others do it. You may want to take driving lessons in order to lean the theory. With constant practice, performance improves. Once you feel comfortable enough, you decide to register for the driver examination which is the definitive test of your ability. The crowning glory is that moment when you sign a driver's permit, signifying a basic level of ability acceptable to the rule makers.

To achieve success requires work. The extent of the work needed is determined in part by your choices and ability. By selecting options that you feel comfortable with, the extent of the work required to achieve success will be less than if you had chosen goals in which you have no interest or for which you have no natural ability. Successful people involve themselves in activities for which they have a keen interest if not a full-blown passion.

Oddly enough, the majority of people I have come across do not feel passionate about their work. Although they have trained and studied for their chosen field or simply have fallen into their line of work, they simply are not fulfilled. Staying in less-than-satisfactory careers is easier and less scary than facing change. Change means uncertainty and unpredictability which, for many, is scary.

The educator with a classroom full of students or the nurse with twenty patients to attend to will likely find the task enjoyable if the work is what makes him or her happy. Difficulties, setbacks, and challenges will be part of their everyday lives but will not hold them back from accomplishing what they have set out to do. In fact, without challenges most activities would be boring. Golfing, for example, considered one of the fastest growing recreational activities, requires practice, commitment, and stamina. Would the game be as interesting if it weren't for sand traps, lagoons, trees, or other obstructions that make the experience more challenging?

Why should you challenge yourself so often? Why is success so important? Success makes a person feel good. The more you feel good, the more you want to accomplish. The more you accomplish, the more you get a sense of personal pride that brings happiness and contentment. The opposite is also true. The less one does, the less one wants to accomplish. This leads to a state of laissez-faire which, in turn, may degenerate into a lack of confidence. Lack of confidence will impact any attempt to accomplish anything and can eventually lead to despair. So in order to succeed, you must never give up on your attempts to make things happen in a winning way.

Everything you do, want, or need falls under the following categories: physical, intellectual, emotional, and spiritual. Together they form the basis or foundation of your existence. If you represent these four categories with a square, you have a framework on which to build. Just as you ensure a solid foundation for your home, you must also have a solid foundation on which to build your life, your dreams, and your successes.

The resultant square is a footing that requires balance. In other words, individuals must take care of their physical, intellectual, emotional and spiritual needs in order to make sure that the foundation of life will not be lopsided. To neglect one aspect or need is tantamount to building on sand. When a house shifts structurally, it is because the foundation is inadequate to support the weight of the house or is built on inadequate soil or sand. Let's continue building the structure by adding triangles on all sides.

I've chosen the triangle since it symbolizes the path to perfection. The bottom of the triangle corresponds to your start in life. At the broadest, the possibilities are huge. You don't yet have a basis for discrimination, thus almost anything, anyone, or any time is acceptable. As time goes on, you learn to reject what you don't like or want and you keep what you enjoy or need.

This process of discarding or shedding is a natural phenomenon. The older and wiser you get, the more you throw away or ignore in favor of what really matters. You realize that you can't be all things to all people, nor do you want to be. Being selective is in fact allowing you to be who you truly are. The same pattern for each of these needs is represented as a triangle. The top of the triangle is the apex, or perfection. Although you never fully realize perfection, you still make daily attempts to improve yourself and avoid making the same mistakes twice. Reaching or aiming toward the higher level of needs (as we discussed earlier when referring to the Clayton Alderfer's ERG Theory) allows you to work toward self-actualization in a way that will bring you closer to fulfilling your own potential.

Adding four triangles to the base will result in a perfect pyramid, one of the world's oldest and strongest structures. With each triangle added to form the pyramid, it becomes clear that each side of the pyramid relies on at least two others, in addition to the base. It is much the same way with needs. Your physical needs would not be complete without emotional and spiritual fulfillment. The extent to which there is interplay between needs is very much dependent on the activity performed and your individual preferences. As no two people are alike, the interactions between needs are very different.

Unlike Maslow's hierarchy of needs, Clayton Alderfer's ERG Theory allows the order of needs to be different for different people. There is also an acknowledgment that if a higher level of needs remains unfulfilled, a person may regress to lower level needs that appear easier to satisfy.

Understanding that experience and wisdom lead to a narrowing of the path reveals why it often takes us a while to figure out our passions. Earlier on in life, you get somewhat confused with all the choices available and, at times, you are influenced by current trends or peer pressure. In staying the course, in due time, what you really are passionate about should surface.

Will that passion lead to success? Is success possible for all of us? You bet!

So before you decide that you can't, ask yourself why not? Everyone knows that you can't achieve success overnight. Yet we often attempt such feats only to fall down. We would be much wiser if we tried to break things into manageable pieces and then attempted to accomplish each in succession. I am reminded of a joke that goes this way. "How do you eat an elephant?" The answer is astonishingly simple: "One morsel at a time."

Nothing challenges me more that someone telling me I can't do this or that. After being told that my life after forty would be spent in a wheelchair, I was determined to do something about it. Although I am not successful with everything I try, I certainly have no fear of attempting even the wildest ideas. Sports people use an expression I find most appropriate: 'a personal best'. In the words of William Faulkner, "Don't just try to be better than critics. Try to be better than yourself." This is what your goals should be, thus raising the bar a little higher but always compared to what you have previously accomplished and not as compared to what others have been able to do. Granted this won't apply to competitive sports where winning is a matter of outperforming the next person. But in most other areas, doing your best will bring success in a way you may not have thought possible. Success brings good health which, in turn, may lead to pain-free living.

An overnight success is hardly done overnight. It has probably taken years of learning and practice to make a person successful. Furthermore, success is not so much a point in time but a way of doing, a way of being. And as with everything else in life, success requires effort, otherwise you can't expect that by sitting on your laurels, success will happen all on its own.

What efforts are required? How do you go about being successful? Remember the four pillars (the walls of the foundation for success)? For each of these, there is a corresponding action that requires your attention on a continual basis. These actions include the following: recognizing and reacting, resting, refueling, and recreating. The following shows the relationship between the pillars and the actions required.

Pillar (needs) (Action)

Physical/emotional/spiritual——··➔(recreating/resting/refueling)

Intellectual (mental)——··➔(recognizing/reacting)

Note that for physical, emotional, and spiritual needs, there is not a one-to-one correspondence with the desired actions. The reason for this is simple. Activities contemplated under refueling, for example, meet more than one need. For example, self-hypnosis is both resting and refueling as it relates to physical and spiritual needs.

The following chart will help you assess your needs. The first column lists three important areas of concern under the four needs (physical, intellectual, emotional, and spiritual) followed by a statement of a specific need to be met. If you agree with the statement, write 'yes'. If not, write 'no'. For each 'no', write a specific action that you could take to address that unmet need. The chart is repeated three times. The first deals with needs with respect to your 'self'. The second chart is for the needs you have with respect to your spouse or partner. The last chart covers your needs with regard to your employer or place of work.

I'm convinced that just ten minutes a day of your time spent on checking your progress with respect to the actions required will ensure success to a degree you would never have dreamed possible. Balancing the five 'R's are a *'sine qua non'* to achieving success.

NEEDS (SELF)

PHYSICAL
Body (I am ok with my body)
Health (I am healthy)
Love (I am content)

INTELLECTUAL
Education (I have the education I need)
Training (I have the training I need)
Challenges (I am challenged and challenge myself)

EMOTIONAL
Security (I feel secure)
Respect (People respect me)
Self-esteem (I have a good self-image)

SPIRITUAL
Religion (I feel free to practice a religion)
Values (I know what's important to me)
Beliefs (I have an established set of beliefs)

NEEDS (RELATIONSHIP WITH SPOUSE)

PHYSICAL
Body (We appreciate each other's body)
Health (We live a healthy lifestyle)
Love (We love each other)

INTELLECTUAL
Education (We have similar educational backgrounds)
Training (We seek training to meet our needs)
Challenges (We decide together the challenges we wish to take on)

EMOTIONAL
Security (We feel secure about our relationship)
Respect (We respect each other)
Self-esteem (We nurture each other)

SPIRITUAL
Religion (We each practice religion our own way)
Values (We share a common vision and values)
Beliefs (We respect each other's beliefs)

NEEDS (WORK/WORK ENVIRONMENT)

PHYSICAL
Body (My body is not an issue)
Health (My health concerns are taken seriously)
Love (My employer understands that I need to balance work life with home life)

INTELLECTUAL
Education (I have the education required to do my job)
Training (I am provided with training as required)
Challenges (I am given interesting and stimulating work)

EMOTIONAL
Security (I feel secure in my work environment)
Respect (My supervisors/colleagues/clients respect me)
Self-esteem (No person does or says things that affect my self-esteem)

SPIRITUAL
Religion (My employer does not discriminate against me because of the way I live my religion)
Values (The values of the organization I work for are congruent with mine)
Beliefs (My supervisors/colleagues/clients do not question my beliefs)

PART 1
Introduction:

In this part of the book, we turn our attention to the physical, emotional, and spiritual dimensions of achieving a drug-free, successful, balanced life. Achieving success with tangible results requires a sound body as well as a sound mind. To neglect either would make the goal of success next to impossible to achieve.

While the second part of this book focuses on the intellectual needs and concerns for achieving health and success, this first part of the book will focus on the physical, emotional, and spiritually needs. Humans have five basic physical needs: breathing, ingestion, digestion, elimination, and exploration. Although you may be aware of these needs, the question is, "What are you doing about them? Are you getting enough sleep? Are you eating properly? Are you exercising regularly? Are you taking time to do the important things in your life?" The answer to these and many other questions concerning your life choices will provide some valuable data on which you can adjust your approach to meet these needs.

A state of well-being is a prerequisite for health and success. Well-being is the opposite of ill-being, and in the words of Lise Bourbeau, "Every state of ill-being is a signal that you are thinking or doing something non beneficial to yourself."[6] I'm not talking about the time when you ate a large piece of cake on a very full stomach. Rather I'm referring to patterns in your ways of doing that indicate negative trends that need your attention. The most common examples of inattention to your physical well-being are overeating, sleep deprivation, alcohol overuse, and inactivity.

This section also deals with emotional and spiritual well-being, which I refer to as 'refueling'. Refueling is the ability to recharge one's batteries through a variety of sources. Recharging can take the form of hobbies, travel, meditation, yoga, prayer, self-hypnosis, visualization, reading for example. There is no cookie-cutter approach that will work for all. So after reading this section, choose those activities that best suit your style and personality and take action.

Grounded individuals achieve a balance between their intellectual and their physical, emotional, and spiritual needs. They most often have an inner peace that is physically apparent, as can be witnessed through the eyes. They smile in ways that say "Hey, I'm happy and I hope you are too."

A 'need' is anything required to sustain life, while a 'want' is anything we wish to have but is not absolutely necessary for daily living. Often we confuse a 'want' for a 'need' and place incredible pressure on ourselves to work harder in order to acquire a 'want'. The more we 'want', the more stress we will endure to obtain these extras. For chronic sufferers, the added stress normally translates into increased levels of pain. Much of this can be avoided by realigning our ratio of 'wants' to 'needs'.

RESTING

Sleeping

"The beginning of health is sleep."[7]
In living a balanced life, one must find time to rest, relax,

and sleep. Getting a good night's rest should not be a luxury, since the body needs to recharge on a regular basis. Without sleep, you are running on an empty tank. For many of us, there is little time to have a full night's sleep. Without adequate sleep, your energy level and desire to succeed are reduced significantly. But what constitutes a full night's sleep? Can that be different for one person than for another?

Some startling statistics have come from organizations such as the National Sleep Foundation, confirming what researchers and industry experts have suspected for years. Fatigue in the workplace costs the American industry at least $77 billion a year. "Employee fatigue has been linked to many of the most notorious incidents of our time, including the Exxon Vadez, Chernobyl, Three Mile Island, not to mention 25 percent of all highway accidents," according to Dr. Martin Moore-Ede, the President and CEO of Circadian Technologies Inc. Recent surveys conducted by Dr. Moore-Ede's team reveal that operations managers believe that employee fatigue is the direct cause of at least 18 percent of all accidents and injuries suffered on the job.

It would be so simple if all you had to do is take a power nap instead of spending hours in bed. However, the body needs deep sleep in order to rejuvenate. Cheating your body of this important source of refueling will certainly lead to health issues. Getting by on minimal sleep will, over time, result in less than stellar work performance, overall irritation, and ill health.

A significant number of people suffer from various sleep disorders including the very common 'sleep apnea'. Sleep apnea is characterized by loud snoring and numerous instances of pauses in breathing during sleep. If you suspect that you suffer from a sleep apnea or any other sleep disorder, you should consult your family doctor for referral to a sleep specialist.

Assuming that you do not have a sleep disorder, the following guidelines will help you get a better night's sleep.

1) Go to bed the same time every day. You will feel better if you eat and sleep at regular times. When your sleep cycle has a regular rhythm, you will be more relaxed. On weekends, try to stick to the same sleep time. However, if that is not possible, take a 20 minute nap before 3:00 p.m. to make up for the lost sleep. If at all possible, rise at the same time the next morning. When you follow a natural sleep rhythm, you will wake up at approximately the same time every day, even if you went to bed later than usual. Avoid naps after 3:00 p.m. or for longer than 20 minutes. As a substitute, try a 20 minute self-hypnosis session discussed in the next chapter of this book.

2) Avoid food prior to bedtime and stay away from caffeine, nicotine and alcohol at least 3-4 hours before bed. In other words, if you eat supper at 6:00 p.m., you should refrain from eating again or taking caffeine, alcohol, or cigarettes between supper and bed time. Caffeine is contained in a variety of products that include coffee, tea, cola, cocoa, chocolate, and some prescription and non-prescription drugs. Products that contain natural sleep inducers such as tryptophan may be taken before bed without problems. Milk contains tryptophan; therefore a warm glass of milk before bed is fine.

3) Avoid exercise at least 3-4 hours before bedtime. Although regular exercise is highly recommended

to help you stay healthy and sleep well, you should exercise in the morning or early afternoon so that it will not interfere with sleep.

4) Before going to bed, take fifteen minutes to wind down from your day's hectic pace. Read, listen to soft music, take a warm bath, do relation exercises, or meditate.

5) Sleep in a cool and quiet bedroom on a comfortable bed with enough layers to stay warm. If you are bothered by early morning light, invest in a blackout shade or wear a slumber mask. If noise is the issue, wear earplugs.

6) If you fail to fall asleep within 20 minutes, get up and sit quietly in soft lighting or in the dark. Read something boring or listen to soft music. Self-hypnosis at this time may be beneficial as well.

Lack of sleep often leads to stress, which in turn leads to ill health. For chronic pain sufferers, sleep is an even more important element in a balanced life. The degree to which pain or discomfort can be handled is often the result of how well a person feels on any given day. While pain management encompasses a number of strategies, there is no denying that the refueling provided by a good night's rest is of paramount importance. At times, the pain is so severe that sleep is affected and in those cases, more attention should be paid to the other strategies contained in the pain management program. Resist the temptation to use drugs, even if it would solve the immediate problem.

The use of medication to ease pain, allowing for adequate sleep, is a tradeoff only you can decide upon. Personally, if my sleep is affected by pain for more than two nights in a row, I consider the impact of not taking some form of medication. In most cases, I will resume medication in half doses to see if I can overcome the problem and get the rest I need. Over time, I have found that I can use medication more effectively if I take it only when I really need it. Since there is no real substitute for sleep, and if all else fails, I must rely on prescription or over-the-counter drugs to tide me over to a better time. Over the years, thanks to a holistic approach to life, I have managed to stay away from drugs two to three years at a time.

"Early to bed and early to rise makes a man healthy, wealthy, and wise."[8]

Self-Hypnosis/Visualizing

"The natural force within each of us is the greatest healer of disease."[9]

Everyone can benefit from learning relaxation methods. Relaxation is the first step in self-hypnosis and meditation. Relaxing helps to reduce stress and ultimately improve your well-being. By using relaxation techniques, you can create your own inner balance and harmony and thus improve your life.

Meditation is a state of relaxation and is an easy way to unwind and to rejuvenate your body. There are numerous physical benefits to be gained from meditation. It can help lower your blood pressure or heart rate. It can help you fall asleep. It can also help reduce stress and stress-related difficulties.

Self-hypnosis is a method of relaxation somewhat similar to meditation. It increases control over the body and mind. Hypnosis is a deeply relaxed state of mind. By instructing your subconscious on modifications you wish to make and behavior patterns you would like to change, through positive constructive suggestions you can bring about beneficial changes to your life. Being in a peaceful trance induced by hypnosis offers you the opportunity to connect with your subconscious and instruct it or reprogram it to follow a new path. Although science has proven that, to some extent, you can control your body, self-hypnosis is most often used to instruct the subconscious to heal, to relax, to find a solution to a problem, or simply to prepare for a very peaceful sleep.

Proper breathing is a prerequisite in using any relation technique. The following steps will help you get there:

1. Take a slow, deep breath for a few seconds and inhale through your nose. Allow the air to expand both stomach and chest taking in as much air as you can.
2. Hold the air for another few seconds.
3. Slowly exhale thought your mouth for 7-8 seconds. Repeat the process, this time noticing the rhythm being created.

Imagine the tension and stress flowing out of your body as you exhale.

Self-hypnosis steps:

Doing self-hypnosis in a quiet place makes it much easier to concentrate and achieve a deeper level of relaxation. With time and practice, you will be able to use self-hypnosis to relax and refresh yourself even in a crowded, noisy bus!

1. Find a quiet place.
2. Find a comfortable position. Lie down and keep your back straight (probably the easiest for beginners).
3. Close your eyes and begin the breaking technique described above. Take several deep breaths followed by deep exhaling.
4. Clear your mind of all thoughts by focusing (and seeing) a candle burning in the centre of an all black room. Once your mind stops racing and focuses on the flame, begin the process of deep relaxation.

The following should either be taped ahead of time and

played when you are ready or read to you in a slow and peaceful voice. Over time, you will be able to memorize the sequence of directions and won't need to rely on a tape or reading. For the first couple of weeks, I suggest that you do at least one session every day until you get the hang of it and until you are able to reach a deep relaxation.

Let us begin to relax.

See the flame.

See the energy from the flame.

Feel the heat from the flame.

Feel the sense of peace at watching the flame and feeling its effects.

Feel the energy provided by the flame.

Feel that energy entering the top of your head.

Feel that energy entering your head and quickly reaching all extremities of your body.

Feel that energy turn into a relaxing power as it starts to move down from the top of your head.

Feel that relaxing power massage your forehead.

Feel that relaxing power massage your eyes.

Feel that relaxing power massage your nose.

Feel that relaxing power massage your mouth.

Feel that relaxing power massage your chin.

Feel that relaxing power massage your neck.

You are beginning to feel great.

You are feeling warm all over.

You are at peace with yourself.

You feel great.

Feel the relaxing power come into your upper arms.

Feel the relaxing power come into your elbows.

Feel the relaxing power come into your lower arms.

Feel the relaxing power come into your wrists.

Feel the relaxing power come into your hands.

You feel great.

You feel warm all over.

You are at peace with yourself.

Your body is getting heavier.

Now feel that relaxing power massage your upper back,
Relaxing each muscle, each vertebra.

Now feel that relaxing power massage your lower back,
Relaxing each muscle, each vertebra.

You feel great.

You feel warm all over.

You are at peace with yourself.

Your body is getting heavier.

You are aware of your surroundings yet you are floating above the noise.

Feel the relaxing power come into your hips.

Feel the relaxing power come into your thighs.

Feel the relaxing power come into your knees.

Feel the relaxing power come into your calves.

Feel the relaxing power come into your ankles.

You feel great.

You feel warm all over.

You are at peace with yourself.

Feel the relaxing power come into your feet.

Feel the relaxing power come into your heels.

Feel the relaxing power come into your arches.

Feel the relaxing power come into your toes.

Feel the relaxing power come into the palm of your feet.

You feel great.

You feel warm all over.

You are at peace with yourself.

(Break here if you want to focus on one item or to use visualization techniques, or to simply fall asleep.)

On the count of five, I want you to open your eyes.

1, coming up, feel the blood coming back to your hands and feet.

2, coming up, feel the blood coming into your arms and legs.

3, coming up, feel a sense of well-being as you begin to awaken.

4, coming up, stretch your arms and legs.

5, open your eyes, open your eyes wide open.

While you may not get enough sleep every night, it is possible to get some form of rest through self-hypnosis. Self-hypnosis is easy and can be used by anyone almost anywhere. Practice makes perfect, and by doing self-hypnosis regularly you will feel recharged, thus giving you a lot more energy.

Self-hypnosis techniques offer a way of reducing pain without taking additional medication. Self-hypnosis has no side effects and will not harm you in any way. As an arthritis sufferer, I can attest to its benefits. Without it, I'm not sure how I would have coped with the horrendous bouts of the disease. Self-hypnosis alone will not cure you of any disease, but is certainly a very useful tool in one's arsenal against chronic pain. Even if you don't have pain, you will discover that self-hypnosis is a remarkably effective way of relieving stress and reducing anxiety.

Visualization techniques or guided imagery can help you overcome mental barriers to success. These techniques provide a way of communication with your subconscious mind. When you 'see' an image or picture in your mind, you are seeing the result of the conscious and subconscious at work.

At the 'break' point in the self-hypnosis procedure,

visualize the necessary steps you will need to take to achieve a particular goal. Once you have done that, visualize the goal as having been achieved. For example, if you wanted to visualize standing up and making a presentation at an AGM (annual general meeting), you might want to start by visualizing yourself writing the speaking notes, reviewing them with a friend, entering the meeting room, being presented, delivering your presentation, taking questions from the audience, and receiving thunderous applause. The visualization need not be very long. Unlike a dream where it feels like being in a movie, visualization tends to be a series of video snippets that run by quite quickly. As you are in control, you can slow down the pace or even rerun a segment of the visualization that seemed out of focus or blurry. Try to focus so that you see very clear pictures of yourself doing what it is that you expect to do. Also important is the approval you get from others at every step of the process.

Visualization is a powerful tool and is used by many successful people. Athletes in particular use the technique to improve their chance of success. However, most people could benefit from the technique if only to help them get some self-assurance. At times, you may feel nervous, doing something you know perfectly well. Visualizing a few hours before the event will likely lessen the stress and make for a smooth and better delivery.

REFUELING

Exercising/getting involved in sports

"The sovereign invigorator of the body is exercise, and of all exercises, walking is the best."[10] Dr. Jarvis observes that "If we would take a leaf out of the animal book we would walk more."

With all the gyms and sports facilities in North America, we should be a very fit society. Yet the rate of obesity is astonishing. You may argue that such facilities cost money and are out of reach to many people. That is true. However, much can be done without incurring any costs at all.

Thomas Jefferson certainly had it right when he suggested that walking is the best exercise. Yet city planners plan and build communities where walking to shops and services is next to impossible. We have come to rely on our mighty automobiles and we use them to get to a gym or sports facility—irony of ironies.

A brisk twenty minute walk every day will offer a cardiovascular workout that's good for what ails you. Walking helps to digest the food you eat. As proper elimination is essential to your well-being, walking should form part of your daily exercise plan. It requires no special equipment or clothing other than good walking shoes to avoid foot and ankle pain.

Daily exercise should be done in the morning or early in the afternoon so as to not interfere with sleep in the evening. As the body ages and stiffens, it becomes important to do a minimum amount of stretching in the morning just after you get out of bed. In fact, you may want to simply remove the covers and do your stretching exercises right there on your bed.

I used to think I had no place in my home to exercise until one day when my physician asked me if I had a bed. "Yes, of course," I replied. "Then you do have a place to exercise," he concluded. With the help of a physiotherapist, I have put together a 45-minute stretching exercise routine which I do religiously every morning. For AS sufferers, early morning stretching is essential to warm up the joints and get the body in shape for the day. Inactivity is what makes joints fuse.

Therefore, limbering up soon after you rise should be part of your daily routine, especially if you have AS or other forms of arthritis.

While being checked by the rheumatologist during my last regular checkup, he noted that, for my age and the number of years I've had ankylosing spondylitis, my mobility is much better than average. I attribute this success, in part, to my determination to exercise on a regular basis.

The added flexibility makes for easier sex. Over the years, I've noticed a great improvement in mobility as a result of my morning stretching routine. Although back problems can provide a convenient excuse to avoid sexual encounters, a regular routine of physical conditioning to tone up your trunk muscles will go a long way in improving your ability to enjoy your partner. In *The Back Doctor*, Dr. Hamilton Hall states: "If you are the one with the back problem, your partner must be patient and understanding, and you should conduct yourself in such a way as to encourage that attitude. Prolonged gentle foreplay, oral sex, and frank conversation can heighten sexual comfort and gratification without adding stress to the spine. You will find that the extra effort required of both of you will be well worthwhile; it will enhance your sex life, improve your marriage, and make your back feel better."

Recent research indicates that as little as fifteen minutes of exercise three times a week will reduce the possibility of Alzheimer's or senility in later years. Any amount of exercise is better than no exercise, so get off your duff and do something. You'll be glad you did!

Eating right

"More die in the United States of too much food than of too little."[11]

Do you eat to live or live to eat? If eating is a real pleasure for you, as it is for me, there are ways to eat and remain healthy. Eating quality food in reasonable amounts at regular times during the day will go a long way toward creating healthy habits and a healthy lifestyle. And in words of Dr. Jarvis, "Good health is earned. In the long run you must pay either the grocer or the drug store."

For most of us in North America, the thought of not having enough food to get through the day is almost unheard of. For most people, the availability of food is not an issue. We live and eat well. However, we eat too much. The most recent statistics point to an ever-growing problem with obesity in the adult population, and of late even in young children. As food is plentiful and very often quite affordable, we tend to eat more than our body needs. Portions have become larger over the years. Witness the ever-increasing popularity of restaurants that serve food buffet style. We are encouraged to eat, eat, and eat. Food advertisements abound on television, in newspapers, in magazines, on the Internet, on billboards, for example. Yet the link between overconsumption and health issues such as type 2 diabetes is seldom made or discussed in the media. Recent research shows a direct link between obesity and type 2 diabetes. That in itself should be enough to stop us right in our tracks at the buffet table. As Peter de Vries so aptly put it in his 1956 book *Comfort Me With Apples*, "Gluttony is an emotional escape, a sign something is eating us."

The adage that says "you are what you eat" holds no new truth but many seem to ignore this truism. It goes without saying that the quality of food you eat has a direct correlation with your level of health. It would be simple if all could follow the same dietary program. But as we all have different health issues, we must find solutions that are tailored to our specific needs and concerns. Regardless of unique needs, our bodies require minerals. Unfortunately, the diet of the average North American is sorely lacking in essential minerals.

At the height of my misery with the arthritic pain, I discovered Dr. Levine, a medical practitioner who told me that my body was full of toxins. He suggested a thorough cleansing of the system by having me abstain from a variety of known irritants such as red meat, caffeine, refined sugar, refined flour, salt, and yeast, to name but the most important. The cleansing process lasted one month, at which time he allowed me to slowly, methodically, be reintroduced to small amounts of the irritant substances. His goal was to rid my body of any substances that caused irritation or inflammation. According to Dr. Levine, keeping such a strict regimen would be very difficult, particularly at first. To make sure I followed his program, he allowed me to disregard the restrictions one day a week. It took about three months for me to feel the difference. But once I did, the level of pain subsided to such an extent that I was convinced of the value of a better diet. Over the years, I have attempted to stick to this regimen. When I follow this dietary approach, I feel better, have more energy, and the bouts of arthritis are much less severe.

You need not have the kind of physical issues I've had to benefit from proper diet. Good eating habits start early and although they may be set aside for a time, particularly in the teen years or while living alone, it is not that difficult to commit to improving one's health, especially when there are payoffs. A diet rich in fruits, vegetables and legumes combined with moderate portions of meat, pasta, fish, bread, cheese, eggs, nuts, and seeds will go a long way toward improving your overall health.

My family doctor, of Chinese origin, suggested to me that

we North Americans typically eat twice the amount of food that is considered sufficient. I took him up on the challenge to reduce by 40—50% all meat and fish portions. The results were almost instantaneous. My digestion improved and I felt much better after leaving the dinner table. Benjamin Franklin believed that "to lengthen thy life, lessen the meals."

Saturated fats (which includes most of our comfort foods such as fries, chips, fried onion rings, etc.), trans fatty acids (which includes most processed food), sugar, caffeine, cream and salt, have no real place in a healthy diet. However, taken occasionally in small amounts will not significantly impact your health. The key is to manage fatty foods with the aim to keep them to a bare minimum. When you have cravings, a good suggestion is to make your own so that you have control over the quality of the ingredients you choose and also on the amount and type of fat you decide to use to make your favorites. For those items you don't care to make, such as potato chips, either buy a small quantity which you can eat at once or buy a larger quantity and set aside a reasonable portion while storing the remainder in a sealed container to be eaten later. Emptying out a huge bag of chips in a large bowl is a good way of making sure that all of it will be eaten. Rather than creating tempting situations, control your portions by putting in front of you reasonable amounts of food to satisfy your craving.

Years ago, I drank on average six to eight cups of caffeinated coffee a day. I enjoyed the boost of energy it provided. But I also knew that I was getting addicted to it. I drank it with 10% cream and lots of sugar. Most of my coffee drinking occurred in the office. I would have a few cups in the early morning to get me going. As the day progressed and most often the stress level increased, so did my consumption of the brew. Typically, by mid afternoon, I was experiencing reflux.

I knew that I needed to address the problem I had created. First, I went to decaffeinated coffee. The withdrawal pains were unbelievable. I had headaches day after day. I reduced my daily coffee intake. However, I still had problems getting rid of the reflux. I needed to find a substitute. When I came to the conclusion that decaffeinated coffee was not an acceptable solution, I switched to hot water with a twist of lemon.

I got a little more creative with my hot water after reading a book written by Dr. D.C. Jarvis entitled *Folk Medicine: A New England almanac of natural health care from a noted Vermont country doctor*. The book extols the virtues of apple cider vinegar[12], potassium, honey, kelp, iodine, castor oil, and corn oil. In his book, Dr. Jarvis claims that apple cider vinegar can be used to treat animals and humans and suggests that a daily intake of apple cider vinegar helps with digestion, eases arthritis and regulates blood pressure.[13] It can be taken undiluted or in a glass of water. As apple cider vinegar is the not the easiest thing to drink[14], the author suggests that it be ingested along with honey, nature's finest ingredient.

Honey is known for its soothing properties (it enters the blood stream quickly and produces a calming effect) and contains more than twenty known minerals. An unexpected benefit was a significant reduction of my eczema. According to Dr. Jarvis, "Honey is not only an excellent food, it is a food supplement too. It prevents fermentation in the gastrointestinal tract and is quickly absorbed. Honey contains important elements for forming new blood. Having a mild laxative effect, it prevents constipation. Being also a body sedative, it helps to produce sound and refreshing sleep."

According to Dr. Jarvis, to be efficient our bodies need minerals. Two good sources of minerals are apple cider vinegar and honey. Dr. Jarvis states that, "In Vermont folk medicine, there is an extremely simple prescription for replenishing the mineral needs of the body. It is as follows: two teaspoonfuls of honey and two teaspoonfuls of apple cider vinegar, taken in a glass of water one or more times each day, depending on how much mental and physical work is done. The blend tastes like a glass of apple cider. The vinegar brings across from the apple its mineral content, the honey brings across the minerals in the nectar of flowers."

Dr. Jarvis makes the case for potassium as an essential for the maintenance of a healthy body. "In humans and animals alike, the body definitely wants potassium and if necessary will go to great lengths to get it." More proof of the benefits of potassium is offered: "Potassium is to soft tissues what calcium is to hard tissues of the body. There is little doubt that potassium slows up the hardening processes that menace the whole blood-vessel system."

On finishing Dr. Jarvis's book, I decided on my 'coffee's permanent replacement', or CPR as I affectionately call it. The recipe is simple.

Coffee's Permanent Replacement (CPR) recipe

In an extra large cup pour in 1-2 tablespoons of Apple Cider Vinegar and one tablespoon of honey.

Add 10-14 ounces of water (warm or hot).

Microwave at high for 1 1/2 minutes for a piping hot early morning drink.

Refrigerate the mixture and serve cold on a hot sunny day.

Makes a wonderful summer drink that children will enjoy.

On days that I feel a cold coming on, I add 1 ml. of Echinacea Herb Tincture to the mixture.

As many office workers do, I used to pick up my coffee and muffin and head off to work. Having given up coffee, I wanted to be able to at least enjoy a good muffin. Most muffins bought in coffee shops are laden with sugar, an irritant I wanted to avoid. Proper digestion being important for me (as it is with most arthritis sufferers), I needed a fiber fix. I searched till I found the perfect solution. Here's my recipe.

Fantastic Fiber Fix muffins (makes 12 small or 10 large)

In a large bowl mix together

1 egg

2/3 cup milk (soy milk also works well)

1/3 cup corn oil (or olive oil)

2 large ripe bananas (ripe bananas can be frozen and used when needed)

2 tablespoons of your favorite low fat/no fat yogurt (optional). Jams can be substituted for the yogurt.

In a second bowl mix the following dry ingredients

1 ½ cup of whole wheat floor (or a blend of corn flour and whole wheat flower)

1 cup of bran

¼ cup wheat germ*

¼ cup ground flax seeds*

½ cup raisins or craisins** (optional)

½ cup walnuts (optional)

1 tablespoon cinnamon

1 tablespoon baking powder

1/3 cup of brown sugar

- *bran can be substituted for the wheat germ and flax seeds
- **dried cranberries

Mix dry ingredients thoroughly and push to sides of bowl. Add liquid mixture in the centre cavity of the dry ingredients and gently fold in until batter is evenly wet. Place in greased muffing tins and bake at 350 degrees F (175 degrees C) for 18-20 minutes or until done.

Note that ripe bananas (going black) can be kept in a freezer and used later. Simply thaw the bananas in a microwave (2 minutes at power level 2 or 20%) or leave on a kitchen counter for 20-30 minutes.

I start every day with my exercise routine followed by breakfast consisting of a glass of my Coffee's Permanent Replacement, a Fantastic Fiber Fix muffin and a banana, orange, or apple.

My temptation to eat potatoes led me to find an alternative that could be either ordered in a restaurant or made at home. I had tried cooking rice on numerous occasions but found that it was a hit or miss affair. One day I stumbled across a 'no fail' rice recipe. I've used this same recipe for more than twenty years. The secret to its success is that you must follow it exactly as written. Once you've made it a few times, you'll get a better feel for making variations.

Charlie's No Fail Rice

Makes four (side) portions. The recipe can be doubled or cut in half simply by doubling or reducing the quantities of liquid and rice. There should always be twice as much liquid as there is rice regardless of the amount of rice to be baked.

Preheat the oven at 325 degrees F (165 degrees C)

In a saucepan, melt, at medium heat, one tablespoon of margarine or butter.

Add 1 teaspoon of herbs (this is where the variations come

in. I typically use basil, dill, and oregano, or any combination thereof. Minced dried onions are also very good).

Pour in one cup of chicken broth. You can make your own, use an OXO cube or something similar. (Once you have mastered the main recipe, you may want to try using beef stock, beef broth, or any fruit or vegetable juice).

Bring to a boil and add ½ cup white rice. Stir.

Bake in an oven at 325 degrees F (165 degrees C) for 20 minutes.

Once cooked, the rice will not clump or stick to the bottom and sides of the pan (If that happens, use a tad more margarine/butter next time). You can get fancy by filling muffin tins with cooked rice and cooling in a refrigerator. Once chilled, turn muffin tin upside down and remove rice cakes. Serve cold or heat up in a microwave. Makes for a great presentation on a dinner plate!

Over the years, I have changed my approach to diet and have focused on my 7/7/7 system, which includes seven foods I try to avoid, seven foods I try to eat as much as I can, and seven food supplements I take on a regular basis. The benefits are not apparent overnight, but in time I began to notice an improvement in my energy level and a reduction in pain and overall discomfort.

Foods to avoid

> Red meat
> Refined white flour
> Refined sugar
> Salt
> Yeast
> Caffeine
> Cream

Foods to increase

Fruit
Vegetables
Legumes
Fish
Honey*
Nuts/seeds
Unsweetened natural juices

* According to Dr. Jarvis, "It is no mere theory but has been proved that bacteria cannot live in the presence of honey for the reason that honey is an excellent source of potassium. The potassium withdraws from the bacteria the moisture which is essential to their very existence." Honey contains numerous minerals including iron, copper, manganese, silica, calcium, potassium, and magnesium. As honey is predigested by the bee, it saves the stomach additional labor. Honey is also known to relieve pain in arthritis.

Food Supplements

Apple Cider Vinegar
Potassium
Kelp*
Alfalfa
Glucosamine
Lecithin
Iodine
* Kelp is an excellent source of potassium

RECREATING

Reading

"Books are nothing but to inspire."[15]

People read because they need to or simply for the joy of it. If your work requires you to read, then reading is a need and not necessarily an enjoyment. Make time to read for the sake of reading. For the sheer fun of escape, nothing beats a good novel. For help with a specific problem, a self-help or how-to book offers useful step-by-step guidelines.

What should you read? Successful people read about successful people. Biographies are a good start. However, biographies tell a story and are not geared to help you learn new concepts. Look for self-help or inspirational books. In the self-help section of your local bookstore, you'll find many 'how-to' books on a plethora of subjects. You may also find books on health issues. In the inspirational section, you will find books that will help you understand more complex and esoteric subjects such as how to cope with loss, grief, stress, or anxiety, for example. You can also find books on reaching happiness, love, joy, balance, good health and satisfying sex.

Other than reading for enjoyment, most people tend to read when there is a need to learn something in particular. It may be connected to one of the elements required to reach the level of success you've set out for yourself or to help you with resting, refueling and recreating. Get into the habit of stopping by your local library or neighborhood bookstore to find those treasures than will help you move your life in the right direction. Reading is not something you can delegate, so if you're not a regular reader, try reading short books that will keep your interest.

If you need to be inspired, look for inspirational books that are specific or general in nature. Books that move us or inspire us may be read cover to cover or simply read by selecting a page at random. In the section entitled 'additional resources' at the end of this book, you will find both types of inspirational reading. A good practice is to leave an inspirational book in a place where you are likely to pick it up regularly and read a few pages. Your night stand might be such a place.

Inspirational books are food for the soul. Don't wait till you're down and out before finding a good source of positive thoughts. Remember that successful people are positive thinkers and, by and large, optimistic. How you get to that level will likely depend on your state of mind and how well things are going for you. To help you cope with the inevitable ups and downs of life, regular inspirational reading is a sure way of keeping you grounded.

Bookstores and libraries have been traditional sources of reading material. However, with the advent of the World Wide Web, electronic books are easily available on a wide variety of topics. Also, ordering books from retailers on the Internet is easy, secure, and convenient.

Reading will help you find ways and means of achieving your goals on the road to success. Setting ten to twenty minutes aside every day to read is a good practice.

"Reading is to the mind what exercise is to the body."[16]

Traveling

"He that travels much, knows much."[17]

To travel is to learn. To travel is to be confronted by ways that are different from your own. In today's business environment, cultivating multiple perspectives is not only a good idea but a must for any company or individual wishing to do business with people from various backgrounds (even right here in North America). Understanding how other people live, work, think, and socialize will provide you with the extra edge needed to be successful. By being respectful and understanding of other cultures, you stand a much better chance to succeed in business.

While it is possible to learn much from reading books, it is easier and much more entertaining to visit people and places and learn first hand why others are different from us. We learn a lot about ourselves when we take the time to visit those parts of the world that are dissimilar to ours. We come back from our journeys with a better understanding of other countries and other cultures but also with a greater appreciation for our own. We take for granted the riches of our industrialized worlds without understanding what it has taken to get us where we are. It only takes a power outage of three to four days for us to be reminded of the comforts to which we have become accustomed.

Successful people have long since found that travel adds to their human dimension. By expanding horizons, by understanding other cultures, you open your mind to new and different ways of saying, doing, feeling, and interpreting. Whether you are in sales, marketing, teaching, engineering, management, or manufacturing, knowledge acquired while traveling can be quite useful in dealing with others.

Unlike business travel, which is most often tiring and does not allow for much time to taste the local flavor, leisure travel allows you an opportunity to learn in a self-setting pace. The type and style of holiday you chose will depend on a number of factors and may include time available, money, climate, solo or group travel, interests, comfort required, security issues, etc. Although you may have a preferred style of travel, choosing a different approach can be very enlightening and you may discover that other modes of travel have benefits you may not have known.

If venturing far from the beaten track makes you feel uneasy, it might be a good idea to travel in an area where you can return home either on the same day or the next day. Take out a map of your area, look at the names of places you have never heard of or names of places you wish to visit, and list a few. Find out what there is to see and do before you arrive at your destination. Internet searches will provide you with a plethora of up-to-date information. Make a plan, budget your expenses, and make a decision on when you want to go.

If doing this kind of travel gives you the comfort level you need to move on to places further afield, then the next time, look for interesting places to visit in your state/province and repeat the same planning steps. The more you travel, the more you will want to travel.

Longer trips will require a bit more planning. You may need to do Internet or library research to find more up-to-date information on your holiday destination.

You can greatly increase your comfort level by taking things from home such a favorite pillow, a stuffed animal, tea bags, special soaps or good luck charms. OBUS forms which can be purchased at your local drug store (pharmacy) provide excellent lumbar and back support. As my back pain subsided considerably, I no longer traveled with my OBUS form. Instead, I took along a small pillow adjusted to ensure proper lumbar support. During winter months, I use a rolled up scarf, which does the trick perfectly.

Whether you travel solo or with others, most forms of vacations fall under one of the following categories: 1) self-arranged; 2) group travel; 3) resort holidays; and 4) cruises. For each of these, there are advantages and disadvantages.

To help you decide on the most appropriate type of holiday,

I have listed advantages and disadvantages (in no particular order) for four types of travel previously mentioned.

Self-arranged holidays

Advantages

Full control of what you want to do and when

Can make any changes you want

Can increase time in one place

Can visit at your own speed

Disadvantages

Can be difficult to budget

Must take the time to plan the trip (research)

Security may be an issue

May have trouble being understood (language)

Pack and unpack at each destination

Group Tours

Advantages

Planning is done for you

Few nasty surprises

Price includes almost everything

Tour guide knows the country, the language

Tour guide provides tips/insights

Can form warm friendships with others in group

Disadvantages

Limited time in each location

Individual freedom is restricted

Pack and unpack at each destination

May waste time waiting for lateness of others

Can be difficult to keep up with the group (physically)

Group may be slowed down by those needing extra walking time

Resort Holidays

<u>Advantages</u>
No need to pack and unpack every day
Normally good and safe food   (4 to 5 star properties normally have several dinning areas)
Evening entertainment included in cost
Safe environment (as well for excursions)
Children may stay free in some resorts
More cost effective if a longer holiday is booked
Properties built with tourism in mind
All-inclusive properties include access to water sports
Costs may include all local alcohol
<u>Disadvantages</u>
Can be costly (particularly in high season)
May not be much to do other than what is included at the resort. Local towns/villages may offer little to outside visitors
Excursions are extras
Resort may not live up to expectations based on brochure photographs
Children may not be allowed

Cruises

<u>Advantages</u>
Hotel follows you (no need to pack and unpack)
Consistently good and safe food
Doctor/nurse on board
Can visit almost any country in the world
Evening entertainment included in cost
Lecturers may be available
May visit 4—5 different countries in a 7—10 day cruise
Safe environment (as well for excursions)

Internet access on most newer cruise ships

Stabilizers ensure smooth sailings

Great for solo travelers (room share programs available on some cruise lines)

<u>Disadvantages</u>

Can be costly (particularly in high season)

Loss time boarding and exiting the ship

Excursions are extras

Ports of call may not be accessible in bad weather

Motion can cause dizziness/sickness (Over the counter Dramamine is often used to alleviate the effects of motion sickness—prolonged use however, may cause internal damage).

Many people fear cruising because they are either afraid of water or afraid to be bored in a confined space. Cruise ships are like floating islands with many of the common amenities that can be found in a resort town. The chances of being bored on a cruise are almost as likely as your chances of going hungry. You can be as busy as you care to be or you can simply find a deck chair to sit, read, and relax in. Since the ship travels mainly at night, most days are spent in ports of call when you can disembark and take in the local flavors. On a typical one week cruise, you are likely to stop at four or five different places allowing you ample opportunity to sample various cultures. As your time in port is usually short (on average six to twelve hours), you can make the best of your available time by booking an excursion. If you book a tour with the ship's Shore Excursion Office, you are guaranteed not to miss the boat when it sails. These short tours will give you a good idea on whether the place (or country) is worth coming back to and spending more time there.

Cruise ships are built to be quite stable and extra precautions are added to make ships even more stable in rough seas. State of the art stabilizers are such that the ship's movement will not likely bother you. It may take a few days to get accustomed to the ever-so-gentle rocking, but most people barely notice it unless the seas swell. Cruise companies do their best to have the ships ply the smoothest waters at the best times of the year. Even during hurricane season, ship captains can normally steer the vessels out of troubled waters or avoid problem areas altogether. An advertised port of call may be cancelled due to the inclement weather.

In the unlikely event that you are affected by seasickness, the crew will provide you with tablets that will really help. As a measure of prevention, some travelers wear the 'behind the ear' patch or motion sickness bracelets. Although the patch is very effective, you should be aware of the side effects, which include dry mouth and a reduction in tear production, causing dry and irritated eyes.

A comprehensive guide for new cruisers is available through most cruise companies. These guides will answer most of the frequently asked questions on cruising. Consult the website of the cruise company you have selected to travel with to obtain an electronic copy of this type of publication.

Tips on packing

For people who travel often, being able to get ready in a jiffy or at the last minute may be crucial. To ease the burden of travel, I recommend the following:

1) Have a prepared list of items or things you normally wear during a trip. From your main list, you can create specific lists for cruise holidays, resort holidays or business travel. You may add or delete items from your list as you use it; however, the task of recalling what you need will be greatly simplified.

Color coordination is a good way of reducing the number of items to pack. Use a two or three-color scheme for maximum mixing and matching. Choose items that can be layered so that you are prepared for an unexpected stretch of cool weather. Items that wash and wear easily are also a sure bet.

2) You can save precious time by having your toiletries bag always ready. Choose a toiletries bag with compartments that allow you to see what is in each. Some of the well-designed bags have an attached strap so that it can be hung on a hook or door handle for greater convenience and less clutter around the sink. Any item that may melt (deodorant sticks, for example) or leak (mouthwash, for example) should be kept in sealed (zip lock) bags.

Medications should be kept in their original containers as customs officers may search your bags. They should be kept in your carry-on luggage for easy access. Should your checked luggage fail to arrive at destination, you may have prevented a very unpleasant situation by having your meds with you in a carry-on bag.

Always have photocopies of your passport and other important cards (medical cards, charge cards, etc.) packed in your luggage. Should you lose any of these items of identification, you will have enough information from the copy to advise proper authorities and the process of obtaining replacements will be speedier.

Identify your luggage clearly as many people travel with very similar travel bags. Use a number of highly visible identification tags bearing your name, address and telephone number. Many people also attach additional markers such as a colored pom-poms or ribbons. Avoid using things that have monetary value or that can be used as toys. These will not likely make the trip since they will be removed by airport baggage handlers. In the event that all identification tags have been torn away, your photocopies of personal identification cards will serve as proof that the luggage belongs to you.

3) If flying, carry-on bags should contain a change of clothing and any medication that you may need while in transit. When cruising, for example, you will not have access to your luggage until it is brought to your state room, which may take some time after you board.

PART 2
RECOGNIZING AND REACTING
Introduction

The link between a healthy lifestyle and success is the key to a balanced life. To focus on one at the expense of the other is a recipe for disaster. Media advertisements extol the virtues of a number of prescription drugs to enhance lifestyle and improve success. Drugs for medicinal or recreational purposes all have side effects with the potential of developing a dependency and rarely do they impact on a person's level of personal success. Rather than using drugs as a crutch to ensure a healthier lifestyle or improve one's lot in life, consider instead a thoughtful approach to life and sustenance.

This section will cover a host of important topics to the achievement of success. Successful individuals share common approaches.

In order for you to move forward with your life, you must take the time to stop and reflect. You must analyze past events and make decisions about the future. Decisions, even important decisions, are made on a regular basis. You use whatever information you have at hand and anything else that you can add to it in order to make informed decisions. In reviewing events that have occurred, it is useful to examine these on the basis of what happened and not what could have happened had a different decision been made. Had I accepted the transfer to

Miami, would I have been promoted sooner? Had I agreed to go on that business trip with my spouse, would I have missed an important club meeting? If you begin to wonder what might have occurred, you will inevitably start to second guess the decisions you're about to make. Second guessing leads to paralysis, which in turn will stifle your ability to lead a successful life. Once you've made a decision, stick with it and allow things to unfold as they should. Allow the unexpected to happen and surprise you and likely it will.

The purpose of this section of the book is to give you more details about the kinds of things you need to consider and what actions you need to take. Success in life is not a matter of getting everything but rather a matter of getting what you need.

If accepting mediocrity is not an option, then read on to find out where you should put your energies.

Goal setting

A goal is the fuel that drives you to achieve. Once you set your goal and begin the journey toward achieving it, you will feel a great sense of pleasure and happiness. This goal should be one of your own choosing. You must decide exactly what it is that you want out of life; no one else can or should decide for you. Although you may take advice from others, the final selection of a goal should be yours. Once you know what you want, you will automatically be connected with like-minded people.

Having a clear goal in mind will allow you to control the direction your life will take. As with most things in life, there is a price to pay. Once you have decided to achieve a specific goal, then resolve to pay that price. Share your goal only with people who are truly interested in helping you. It's always a good idea to write down the goal and add to it a visual that depicts the attainment of it. The picture should contain an image of you doing or being what it is that you want to achieve. This picture can then be transferred to a mental image which you can refer to on a daily basis to remind yourself of what is it exactly that you want to achieve. This (mental) image can be used during self-hypnosis as well.

My goal is _____

_____.

Paste a picture of yourself achieving this goal here.

A goal may be specific or general in nature. If your goal is a safari in Kenya, then your visual could contain a scene from a game reserve. You might be sitting in a jeep observing wildlife. If your goal is more general, such as the Director of some large human resources department, then your visual could be a picture of you in a large corner office with lots of files and people coming in and out.

In addition to the mental visual, the actual composite ought to be put in a place where you are likely to see it several times a day. For most people, the refrigerator door is a sure bet.

You may have several goals you would like to achieve, some specific and others more general. The extent to which you can establish goals and the detailed plans that will inevitably need to be hatched to achieve them is a measure of your skill to reach success.

Success will occur at every step of the way if you stay focused on what you want and adjust to changing circumstances and conditions. Nothing is more enjoyable than making small but surely good progress toward a goal. The sense of moving in the right direction will fuel you to keep going and to stay on track.

Winning an Olympic medal is a good example of a specific goal that many aspire to. To get there, an athlete must be willing to work hard, be dedicated, and stay focused. Staying focused, practicing, and getting outside help to improve performance will go a long way toward achieving the stated goal. Accidents will create road blocks or setbacks that need to be dealt with. These may lead to a modification of the original goal or to the establishment of new goals.

A good example of a setback that would have changed a person's goal was typified in the late Christopher Reeve. His fall from a horse left him quadriplegic and created a major setback. Whatever plans he had at the time that required full body ability had to be shelved. He realigned his priorities and set new goals. His determination to succeed despite all odds was exemplary.

Although your setbacks may not be as dramatic as what was experienced by Reeve, they will occur and you will need to deal with them. The unplanned and unexpected often make us change a set course of action. While you have no control over such situations, your ability to readjust when necessary is another mark of your ability to succeed.

The most memorable expression of goal setting is captured in the following question and answer. A music student in New

York stops a local resident and asks how to get to Carnegie Hall. The response is fast and simple: "practice, practice, practice." And so it is with life goals. Nothing will replace hard work and dedication. Hard work and dedication will be all for not if there isn't a clear goal in mind.

If your goals don't move, inspire, or excite you, then you have not found the right ones.

Objectives

Objectives are the milestones along the way. Say you decide to travel from Montreal to Miami. Your goal is to drive to Miami in three days or less. Your objective might be to reach Virginia by the end of day one and Georgia by the end of day two, leaving you with less than a full day's driving on your third and last day. You may also have other objectives, such as getting to the destination without incident or accident. Stopping every two hours could be another objective.

As you achieve each objective, you have succeeded in meeting a planned target. Establishing objectives in support of goals is a way of ensuring that bite-size pieces of the journey can be done without giving up hope. Tackling a goal is daunting at best. Breaking it down into manageable components makes it easier to stay focused and to achieve.

There is no set number of objectives to establish. Some goals may require more, some less. And as with goals, the unexpected and the unplanned can throw a loop into your plans. When these occur, you must take time to analyze what is happening and decide on an alternative course of action. Say you reach the outskirts of Washington, D.C. and there is a roadblock. Cars are getting through but at a snail's pace and you have been caught in traffic for twenty minutes. You assess the situation and look at your maps. Should you leave the highway at the next exit or should you stay on the road in the hope of getting past the roadblock in a reasonable amount of time? You had planned on stopping for a picnic dinner on the south side of the city. Since you're moving so slowly, should you perhaps eat your food in the car and forgo the planned stop so that you can make your first day's objective?

No one can tell you what you should do. It's up to you to analyze, review, and decide once a setback occurs. Some setbacks will have little impact. Had you decided to eat in the car and kept on driving to meet your first day's objectives, the impact would have been minor. Had you decided to leave the interstate at the next exit and tried to find an alternative route, chances are you would have either taken longer to reach the planned stop on day one or, worse, you may have gotten lost and decided to take a room in the first hotel you spot, leaving you the option of going back to the same interstate you left earlier.

Writing down your objectives for such a trip may be somewhat overzealous. Doing so when it comes to your life plans is another matter altogether. The longer the journey, the better the chances you have of staying on top of things and checking progress if you have written down your objectives. Being slightly off course may not be entirely bad, but knowing that you are slightly adrift gives you an opportunity to decide whether you want to make changes.

Side roads can be delightful. You can experience things you would have missed on the highway. Likewise, life tangents are either a welcomed divergence or an annoyance you could do without. If you are the type of person who allows for the unplanned, benefits may come your way. The serendipitous nature of our lives helps us accept the unexpected or fear it.

There are many roads that lead to Rome, all of which include a host of pleasant and unpleasant experiences. As nothing is perfect, going with the flow will help you remain calm. That is not to say that you shouldn't be on your guard at all times, but you should be open to events, people and things that you had not considered. These may help you reshape your objectives in a manner you never thought possible.

List three to five goals in support of your stated objective:

1. _____
2. _____
3. _____
4. _____
5. _____

Competence and confidence

"Who has self-confidence will lead the rest."[18]

Success requires competence. Competence starts with feeling capable in what you do. How do you measure up? How do others see you? Can you consider yourself a success in any one area or field of work?

Many people do not believe that they are good at what they do, even when told so by others. Self-doubts are powerful and often override facts that point to contrary evidence. Combined with second-guessing, self-doubts can lead a person to intellectual paralysis.

Does competence or confidence come first? To succeed, you will need a certain amount of confidence. You can build your confidence in small increments at a time. The more confidence you have, the greater the self-esteem. Strong confidence and good self-esteem will pave the way for competence. As you improve with every attempt, your confidence will increase and your level of competence will be similarly effected.

Let's suppose you decide to take up ballroom dancing. You need the courage to call or visit a ballroom dancing school. You may have very little competence in any form of dancing, but you have confidence that you can learn given the right environment. You register and attend the first class. The instructor comments positively on your limited competence in order to build up your confidence. At first, the lessons will be private so that you can learn the basics and gain a degree of confidence in your own ability. Later an invitation will come to a group lesson or evening social where other students, accompanied by their instructors, will dance newly-learned steps. To be able to cope with the increased pressure of a group situation, you will need to increase your confidence by practicing various dance patterns with a variety of partners.

Confidence will impact everything you do in a positive fashion. Without it, you may feel that doubt undermines your every move. Lack of confidence will lead to fear of performing tasks or activities. Should fear set in, consider going back to the types of activities you do best, in order to regain confidence, and then try again later to accomplish more challenging tasks.

Confident individuals look to successful people for insight and inspiration. They carefully study how these individuals succeed. They are curious about how successful people have overcome the inevitable obstacles of life.

To succeed means making choices and the choices should focus on those things for which you have a natural ability or can easily pick up. Thus, you can move quickly to become extremely competent, which will do wonders for your confidence. You will need confidence to bring your skills up to the next levels.

Being an expert in any one field requires you to commit

to one area of knowledge or ability at the expense of others. However, the advantages of being an expert are that people will seek you out for your opinions and perspectives because they have less knowledge and expertise in a given area. Likewise, you will call upon others for information in areas where they have a much higher degree of expertise.

There is no better way of becoming invaluable to an organization than developing expertise and making it available to others. People will seek your wise counsel and respect and follow your suggestions. You will have achieved competence and will reap its rewards. Be aware that competence in some fields is rather fleeting. Failure to continue to read up and be informed of changes in your field of interest will render you stale rather quickly. This often happens to people who retire and decide that they no longer want to maintain their level of expertise. The old maxim of 'use or lose it' applies.

Competence requires that you use your intellectual abilities, and many studies have proven that when a person reduces intellectual activities, his or her abilities are consequently affected. With the decrease of mental agility usually comes a corresponding decline in health. A 'couch potato' can get up and do either stimulating activities or become 'mashed potato'.

Don't spread yourself too thin. Try not to claim too many areas of expertise. Such attempts can only lead to loss of confidence as you try to keep up in each area. Ultimately, these failures will be reflected by a corresponding loss of self-confidence, which is very self-defeating.

"They can do all because they think they can."[19]

List three to five areas of competence:

1. _____
2. _____
3. _____

4. _____

5. _____

Passion and motivation

"Only passions, great passions, can elevate the soul to great things."[20]

Passion is the intense and unrelenting interest or ability to believe or to do one thing over the other. Passion usually drives a person to excellence. Blood is to the body what passion is to the soul. While reason is linked to logic, passion comes from emotions. There is no right or wrong when it comes to passion. You either have a passion or don't. To have passion is to have a vision of what it is you want.

Passions come from your personality. If you are uncertain as to your personality type is, you may want to seek out people who administer the Myers-Briggs or Strong-Campbell evaluations. Consult career advisors or counselors at your workplace or ask your doctor to suggest the name of a firm in your area that does this type of testing.

Smart people choose activities or jobs based on their personality traits and thus on their passions. Introverts and extroverts will not likely find the same set of duties challenging. The extrovert looks for situations where they can interact with others while the introvert might feel quite a home in a library putting books back on the shelves or developing code for a software program.

There are many personality types and, for each, there is a profile that will help you understand what moves you. Over the years, your personality may change slightly as events unfold in your life. But by and large, people remain relatively constant. Knowing who you are and what makes you happy is the first step toward finding your passion.

Passion should come naturally. It's not something that someone can force on you no more than you would force yourself to like opera. It should come from within, from the heart, and should reflect your true personality. Remember, you will never regret what you do when it comes from the heart; you'll regret what you didn't do.

Passion is our basis for motivation. People who enjoy their work do it better because they care about the results. Why should you care? Successful people care about what they do because each outcome reflects who they are and how they are perceived. In business, perception is nine-tenths of success. If people perceive you as successful, then you will be a success. On the other hand, if you are perceived to be unconcerned about results and about the perception of others, you will not likely enjoy a high degree of success.

Motivation is fueled by your degree of competitiveness. Winning at all costs is not advocated but rather a healthy dose of competitiveness. Competitiveness reflects a desire to succeed, whatever your reason is for wanting it. Nobody can motivate you. Only you can motivate yourself. You can be inspired by others to act. Reading an inspirational book or hearing a good speaker or preacher might move you. In the end, you alone will decide whether or not to act on what you have learned.

The vast majority of people work in jobs they do not enjoy and for which they have no passion. The result is poor performance or shoddy products. Why would you stay in a job that doesn't reflect who you are? The grumpy server who throws food at customers is not happy about being there and is not creating a happy atmosphere for those in the restaurant. The results can damage the bottom line and the reputation of the establishment, to say nothing of the impact to the self-esteem of the individual.

People tend to take their jobs home with them when they leave their place of work. Low satisfaction on the job can be linked to lack of overall enjoyment in life. Over time, family life and health will be affected. It is best to keep your work life and family life apart. That doesn't mean that you shouldn't talk about work while you're at home or vice versa, but you should not take your troubles along with you when you move from one to the other. A good way of achieving this is to bathe and change clothing when you get home from work. Tell yourself as you come to the door that you are leaving your work problems outside the house. Once refreshed after a soothing shower or bath and a change of clothes, you will feel much better and the transition will be much easier.

Apart from sleeping, the time spent at work is greater than the total time taken for all other activities combined. It becomes obvious that work defines who you are to a large extent. So why would you not want to focus on the types of work that truly stimulates you, particularly if you are in a job that doesn't give you the kind of satisfaction you want?

Think about the types of activities, tasks, or jobs that give you fulfillment. Can you find a job where you can perform those skills? If not, starting a new business might be the right answer. Many people have started home-based businesses that have come from personal interests. As the baby boom generation leaves the workforce, many are turning to self employment using skills they really enjoy.

Finding your passion will lead to competence and confidence and is a sure recipe for success. Whether you work for yourself or for a company, having passion for what you do will bring a measure of success. Once you attain higher levels of success, you will crave even more successes. The danger is in letting success be the only value you hold dear. Be passionate about what you do so that you can be successful, but balance that with other aspects of your life, including refueling, recreating, and resting.

"If you can fall in love with what you are doing, it will propel you like nothing else. Vision in life is the most powerful thing in the world. It attracts you in a way that no ambition or plans can ever do."[21]

From the areas of competence you listed in the previous chapter, what are the areas you are most passionate about?

1. _____

2. _____

Fear and setbacks

'If we let things terrify us, life will not be worth living."[22]

From a very young age, your parents taught you to be careful about certain things, situations, or people. For example, you have probably been told not to touch the stove when it's hot. Slowly you have internalized what you can do and what you shouldn't. The line between what is doable and what you should avoid becomes blurred with time. As a teenager, you begin to challenge your parents' interpretation of what's right and wrong. Although they were trying to help guide your life, they may have inadvertently transferred to you some of their fears.

It is hard to imagine a situation where a parent did not influence a child to a great extent. A mother who has a fear of water because one of her siblings downed may want to ensure that her child learns to swim and not be afraid of water despite her own phobia. The reality is that in most cases the child will pick up the subconscious or unstated feelings of the parent. Parents try hard to protect and shield their children from unpleasant experiences, but it is through trial and error that children and adults learn. To be afraid to do something because it may not turn out the way you want is depriving you from many solid learning experiences.

As children often imitate their parents, they may develop patterns of fear or simply a defense mechanism for avoiding doing something that they think they cannot do perfectly. Some children grow up placing limits on what they believe they can accomplish. Adults do this as well. The only real limits are those you place on yourself. You can overcome your fears by getting rid of your old ways of thinking. You must be willing to adopt a 'can do' attitude in order to succeed.

Overcoming fear will not happen overnight. Once you've identified a fear and you are determined to overcome it, you will need to find ways to challenge yourself. One of my greatest fears (and I still have it today) is being under water. The mother I spoke about earlier in this chapter is mine. I can't remember the exact moment I started fearing water but I do recall having shortness of breath when my mother would put my head under the tap to wash my hair. Later, swimming lessons proved to be disastrous. For years, I simply avoided water other than to bathe. During my teens, I was in a boarding school for two years. Showers were the only option and I learned to get over my fear of water cascading over my body simply by getting into the shower every morning. Years later, I was able to enjoy being under water in a shallow pool. Buoyed by that level of confidence, I used flotation devices to move to the deep end of the pool. Today I travel on cruise ships, play in the middle of the lake at the cottage (albeit with a life vest) and enjoy water for the soothing pleasures it offers.

The time you spend worrying about things that could go wrong is time that could be used to improve. It follows that worrying about things that may go wrong increases the chance that they will. Simply accept that sometimes things will work out and sometimes not. The time you save by not dwelling on the possibility of failure is time you can use to think about the many things you can achieve.

Obviously, you can never fail if you don't try. Not trying is, in fact, the greatest failure of all since you will never be able to attain your objectives or reach your goals. The fear of failure can paralyze even the smartest amongst us. Yet, fear itself can be a motivator since people typically don't admit to others that they feel incapable of doing this or that. Taking baby steps in the right direction is better than doing nothing at all. By gaining momentum and confidence, you will acquire competence over a period of time.

A certain degree of fear can be helpful in that it may steer you away from foolish endeavors. This level of fear is at the bottom end of the spectrum and equates to caution, which is something you will need to be successful. Caution in all of your affairs, whether in business, at home, or at play will serve you well. And as Confucius once stated, "The cautious seldom err."

While caution will help keep you in good stead, you are likely to suffer setbacks on the journey to success. Regardless of why setbacks occur, they present a golden opportunity for you to learn. In fact, in reviewing why things got derailed, you may discover what led you to the choices you've made. Have you in fact chosen a goal that is consistent with you, with your values? Do you derive enjoyment and excitement from your choices? Is it in step with what you want to achieve in the long run? Is it a stepping stone to get to where you want to go? Every time setbacks occur, ask yourself these questions. The answers to these should give you a good indication of whether or not you're on the right track. If you are, then the setback is simply life's way of letting you know that you have something to learn from the situation. If you're not on the right track for success, then you may want to reconsider your goal and readjust accordingly.

All throughout high school, my goal was to become a world class interior designer. I had selected this goal based on my passion for design, my interest in the profession, and my personality. An "interest test" given to me by the school Guidance Counselor had clearly shown that of all professions, I had the greatest chance of success in the field of interior decorating. I set out to select the best Interior Design school I should attend. To meet the entrance requirements, I needed to have completed Grade 13. As I was living in a province where this level of education did not exist in the school system, I opted for going to college for a year which would meet the requirement. At the end of year, I was appalled when I discovered that I had failed miserably and would not be admitted to the Design school. It was a setback that left me reeling for years. It took me at least another two years to find something else to replace my initial choice, something about which I could be passionate.

A change of goals is a major setback but need not be the end of your successes. In fact, the tangent I took led me to very different kinds of choices that have worked well for me. While waiting to find suitable employment after my disastrous first year of university, I spent time at home completing a very elementary 'Introduction to Interior Decorating' course from a correspondence school. Fourteen years later, needing extra money to meet mortgage payments on my first house, I started a home-based interior decorating consulting business.

Fear and setbacks are part of life but shouldn't hold you back. Learn to master your fears so that they don't stop you from achieving what you are capable of. When things don't go your way, try gaining something positive from these situations every time they occur.

Luck and Happenstance

"Chance favors the prepared mind."[23]

To a great extent, chance is what you make of it. Once a person achieves a certain degree of success, others will be tempted to say that the person is lucky. Indeed the person is fortunate to have succeeded, but success did not come merely because of luck or happenstance. Luck or opportunity may have played a key role in your success but, in the final analysis, you will come to realize that many other elements came into play, including timing, stamina, persistence, knowledge, networking, and originality.

There is an element of chance in everything. Quirks of fate have had an impact on just about everything that has happened to you since you were born. Great opportunities are to be found every day by those who take the time to look for them. When you are ready to move forward, your mind and your eyes open up to absorb information around you. You open the newspaper to find the perfect opportunity or the perfect job. You talk to a stranger on a bus who tells you about a friend who is looking for a partner to launch a new venture. You attend the funeral of an office colleague and get introduced to someone who shares your passion for the food and beverage industry. Is this luck, happenstance, or fate? What is important is that you pay attention to any and all information that can help you achieve your goal. Carry a journal or agenda and write down important information, such as names and locations of good contacts, useful telephone numbers, and email addresses, quotations, information sources or pearls of wisdom. You'll never know when these may become useful and you'll be happy to have stored the information for later use.

On any given day, chance will play for or against you. As you can't be sure of outcomes, you can nevertheless be open to what comes your way. By trying, you have a 50% chance of success. Either you succeed or you don't. The more you try, the greater the chance you have of hitting the target. The odds are that those who try and try again will likely achieve success. Those who fail to try will simply fade away.

Abraham Lincoln once said that "People are just about as happy as they make up their minds to be." By replacing 'happy' with the word 'luck', the same holds true. People are, in fact, just about as lucky as they make up their minds to be. Having a winning attitude will lead to many lucky breaks. Other than games of chance, luck is the residue of good design, of a good plan. Good fortune is often a question of hard work. The harder you work, the luckier you get.

Luck is also a matter of opportunity. And in the words of Demosthenes, a Greek philosopher, "Small opportunities are often the beginning of great enterprises." Being at the right place at the right time is fortuitous. If you believe that good things will come to you, you need to get out there and be seen so that when opportunity presents itself, you may be the one to benefit from it. Imagine what would happen to a business person who was afraid to leave the office! How many golden opportunities would be missed by not going out and meeting potential clients, business associates or competitors?

As I mentioned previously, things have a way of happening that can be rather annoying at the time until you realize why your plans didn't materialize. Someone or something else gets in the way but ends up being of great benefit to you.

Time and timing

"Hard work means prosperity, only a fool idles away his time."[24]

Carpe diem. Seize the day. A day goes by in a flash. Unless you plan your day, you are likely to waste 20 to 50% of your time on useless or insignificant matters. As you get older, time goes by even faster. Time can neither be saved nor retrieved. Although the focus of this book is not on accumulating a fortune, "time is money."[25] It is a precious commodity that needs to be carefully managed; otherwise it will evaporate, leaving you with nothing to show for.

Unlike a budget where you account for dollars and cents, time is more than simply an accounting of minutes in a day. What you do with your time is as important as the quantity of time available to you. By using time more effectively, you can get more things done. Time management tools, training, and aids can be of great help in improving your use of this limited commodity.

Probably the majority of people would welcome more time to do the things they want to accomplish. The key to time management is deciding what is important and what is not. As you have a limited number of hours at your disposal in a day, the allocation of time to various activities will be an indication of the importance you attach to each. Sleep and work account for the largest chunk of time, leaving precious little for all of the other important things that need to get done. One of your measures of success will be how well you can balance your time commitments, particularly those over which you have a greater say.

Successful people are those who have mastered the art of time management. The notion of successful time management will apply in your work life as well as your home life. However, it is not the time you spend thinking about work or family that will lead to satisfaction but rather the quality of those hours where you do great work or care for your loved ones at home.

It is my belief that a successful day includes time spent on the four "R's" as mentioned in 'Getting Started'. Each day should have its share of: recognizing & reacting (work), resting (sleep, relaxation), recreating (fitness, sports, hobbies, and interests) and refueling (food for the body and soul). The proportion of these four types of action will vary from one day to the next. Failure to consider and include each type in your daily life will lead to an imbalance.

Timing is the ability to do or say the right thing at the right time. Great timing comes with practice, persistence, and observation. Observe what happens around you and take mental notes of what occurs. Pick up on nonverbal cues and clues. Size up people who you intend to deal with. Find out what makes them tick, what's important to them, their likes and dislikes. The more you know about the people around you, the better your chance of good timing. For example, if you knew that Mary's mother had just passed away because you keep up with her, you would instinctively know that now would not be a good time to pitch a new idea or concept or discuss your plans for merging. Conversely, if you had picked up on the fact that

Bob likes baseball, you could invite him to a game and discuss business at an opportune time.

"I must govern the clock, not be governed by it."[26]

"A stitch in time saves nine."[27]

FINAL WORDS

I believe it was my determination to find long-lasting relief to my chronic pain that sent me on a journey of discovery and self-discovery. I discovered that the side effects and the effects of long-term use of prescriptions drugs were simply unacceptable to me. I also discovered that my ability to lead a successful life was directly linked to my well being and that the former goes hand in hand with the latter.

Through trial and error, I was able to rid myself of chronic pain, which allowed me to pursue excellence and success. In attempting to reach success, I discovered that finding my passions in life led directly to less stressful home and work situations, which in turn had positive impacts on my health. It was then that I concluded that health and success are inextricably linked.

On my path to success, I read many books that helped me shape the way I see and define success. The majority of works I read made no link between health and success. For many, health is not a big issue in their lives, or at least not in their early years. Not so in my case. I was determined to reduce chronic pain and be successful. The road I took was one that wasn't clearly indicated. I had to take many side roads, to experiment and experience with new concepts and take a plunge into unknown areas.

The result is that I'm beating the odds. I would be remiss if I left this world without sharing what I've learned.

Obviously, there is no scientific breakthrough here but simply a discussion of a holistic approach to life. If it worked for me, I'm convinced it can help others. The more successful people out there, the better this world will be. Don't expect to have it happen overnight!

You can be born a millionaire, but to be successful you will need to work at it. The path to success is a life-long journey. Success is much more than having possessions; it is living a life of contentment (including health), doing what you enjoy the most, what you are passionate about. Finding your passion and what to do when you've made that discovery is the first step toward improving your life.

Few are those who quickly find their passions, their reasons to live. Many try different things in the hope of finding that particular gift that makes them special, a gift that can be shared and put to good use. Our gifts, used wisely, can yield both tangible and intangible results. While money and worldly possessions are useful, in and of themselves, they do not make a person entirely successful or healthy. What makes a successful person is that delicate balance or mix of health, skills, happiness, contentment, self-sufficiency, self-satisfaction, and love.

To achieve this difficult balancing act requires time and perseverance. Remember the four "R's" that require your regular attention: recognizing and reacting, resting, recreating, and refueling. By constantly monitoring your progress against stated objectives, you will be in a better position to know what needs to be done in order to achieve health and success.

At all times, trust fate. Life has a way of putting onto your path the people and things you need and, at the appropriate time, removing obstacles that are in your way. The more you believe that things happen for a reason, the more you will begin to look for those reasons and learn from them. Remember also that 'What goes around comes around'. What you do to others will someday be done onto you. Just look around and notice those who have fallen and why it happened. Treat others as you would like to be treated and you'll start noticing how much easier life gets. People will cooperate with you, people will do business with you, people with share trade secrets with you—but only if you deserve their respect.

Nothing will change until you decide to make it happen. To achieve your goals, you need to try. If you don't try, you'll have no chance to succeed. In the words of US President Franklin Roosevelt, "It is common sense to take a method and try it. If it fails, admit it frankly and try another. But above all, try something."

It is impossible to know everything before trying something. Sometimes, going on blind faith may be valid. Although you will regret bad decisions, it is fear of regrets that stifles your growth. A Middle East fable tells the story of travelers arriving at a remote oasis in the desert. Just as they were getting ready to lie down for the night, they heard a voice: "Fill your pockets with sand. Tomorrow you will be happy and sad about it." Although skeptical, they followed the order and filled their pockets before going to sleep. The next morning to their surprise and amazement, they discovered that through the night the sand had been transformed into precious stones. They jumped with joy until one of them started to regret not having put more sand in his pockets. Then they all felt sad and were annoyed at not having been told by the voice that such a miracle was about to happen. Had they known, they would all have put more sand in their pockets.

How much sand will you put in your pockets? What actions will you take as a result of reading this book? For each action, set a realistic start and end date and track your progress on a weekly basis.

With respect to my physical needs, I will:

1. _____
2. _____
3. _____
4. _____
5. _____

With respect to my intellectual needs, I will:

6. _____
7. _____
8. _____
9. _____
10. _____

With respect to my emotional needs, I will:

11. _____
12. _____
13. _____
14. _____
15. _____

With respect to my spiritual needs, I will:

16. _____
17. _____
18. _____
19. _____
20. _____

Should you choose to share with me your struggles to improve your health, you can write me at charo@sympatico. ca.

ADDITIONAL RESOURCES

The following books have had a huge impact on my life and have helped me to live drug-free and to succeed in ways I could not have imagined.

1. *Folk Medicine: A New England almanac of natural health care from a noted Vermont country doctor* (D.C. Jarvis, M.D.)
2. *The Back Doctor* (Dr. Hamilton Hall)
3. *The Complete Guide to Nutritional Supplements* (Brenda D. Adderly)
4. *Listen (to your best friend) Your Body* (Lise Bourbeau)
5. *The Power of Positive Thinking* (Dr. Norman Vincent Peale)
6. *Leadership and the One Minute Manager: Increasing Effectiveness Through Situational Leadership* (Ken Blanchard & Patricia Zigarmi)
7. *The Wealthy Barber* (David Chilton)
8. *The Millionaire Next Door* (Thomas J. Stanley & William D. Danko)
9. *How to Read a Person Like a Book* (Gerard I. Nierenberg)
10. *The Road Less Travelled* (Scott Peck)
11. *The Little Prince* (Antoine de St. Exupéry)
12. *Life Little Instruction Book* (H. Jackson Brown Jr.)
13. *All I Need to Know I Learned in Kindergarten* (Robert Fulghum)

14. *The Magic of Believing* (Claude M. Bristol)
15. *Jonathan Livingston Seagull* (Richard Bach)
16. *The Phantom Tollbooth* (Norton Juster)

ABOUT THE AUTHOR

Charles Seems was born in Dalhousie, N.B. (Canada) in September 1952 of an American Father and French Canadian (Acadian) Mother. He graduated from the Université de Moncton in 1976 where he earned a Bachelor of Translation & Interpretation degree. He moved to Ottawa where he taught French as a Second Language in West Quebec schools. He earned a Certificate of Teaching French as a Second Language from the Université du Québec in Hull in 1978 and a Bachelor of Education from the University of Ottawa in 1980. Charles is the author of the Collection Turlututu, a collection of 16 (French) phonetic books for primary grades and the Collection Parminou, a collection of four bilingual (French-English) books for preschoolers. He has published selected poems in Éloizes, a French Canadian literary quarterly.

Charles joined the Federal Public Service of Canada in 1981 and resigned in 2002 having worked in management and human resources consulting for 21 years. In 1986, Charles founded 'Interiors by Design' a residential interior decorating consulting business. In 2002, he launched HR Spectrum offering HR training, coaching, tutoring and consulting services to Canadian federal government departments.

Over the years, Charles has worked in the banking sector, in the hospitality industry, in the education sector, in management consulting, in human resources consulting and in interior decorating consulting. Charles shares his life with his spouse Robert Labine Jr.

You can reach Charles Seems at charo@sympatico.ca.

HEALTHY SUCCESSFUL PEOPLE MAKE SUCCESSFUL BUSINESSES

B ook Charles Seems to speak at your next meeting or event.

Charles conducts his flagship presentation 'Cruising to Success' for managers that want to help employees succeed and businesses that want to increase productivity and improve their bottom line. Depending on your format, time available and meeting objectives, his presentation can be tailored to run from thirty minutes to three hours. It focuses on the relationship between the requirements of a business and the needs of employees leading to successful employees, better employee/employer relationship, better products/services and thus more profits.

For booking information, you can reach Charles directly at (613) 237-3580 or at <u>charo@sympatico.ca</u>.

END NOTES

[1] Ralph Waldo Emerson
[2] David Niven, The 100 Simple Secrets of Successful People
[3] Henry David Thoreau
[4] Where the Blue Begins, 1922
[5] Mark Twain, Letter to Mrs. Foote, Dec. 2, 1887.
[6] Listen (to your best friend) Your Body, Éditions ETC, 1989.
[7] Anonymous (Irish Proverb)
[8] Benjamin Franklin
[9] Hippocrates
[10] Thomas Jefferson, Letter to Thomas Mann Randolph, Jr., Aug. 27, 1786
[11] John Kenneth Galbraith, The Affluent Society, 1958
[12] Vinegar has been used in one form or another for over 10,000 years. It is currently used for many purposes and throughout the ages has served as a preservative, condiment, beauty aid, cleaning agent and medicine. The ancient Egyptians are commonly recognized as the inventors of apple cider vinegar, or at least they were the first to realize its medical benefits. Records show that as far back as 3000 BC, the Egyptians were using apple cider vinegar not just as an antiseptic, but as a weight loss agent as well.
[13] For the benefits of cider vinegar: http://www.lacetoleather.com/wondrugpag3.html
[14] Although apple cider vinegar is available in pill form, I prefer to use the liquid form.
[15] Ralph Waldo Emerson, The American Scholar, 1837

[16] Richard Steele, The Tatler, Mar. 18, 1710

[17] Thomas Fuller, Gnomologia, 1732

[18] HORACE, Epistles, 20-8 B.C.

[19] VIRGIL, Aeneid, c. 19 B.C.

[20] DENIS DIDEROT, Discours sur la poésie dramatique, 1773-78

[21] Leaving a Lasting Legacy (Cavett Robert, NSA)

[22] SENECA, Epistles, 1st cent. A.D.

[23] Louis Pasteur, Speech, Dec. 7, 1854

[24] King Solomon's Book of Proverbs (28:12)

[25] Benjamin Franklin, Advice to Young Tradesman, 1748

[26] GOLDA MEIR, quoted in Oriana Fallaci, L'Europeo, 1976

[27] Anonymous proverb